Digital Hearing Aids

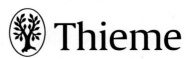

Digital Hearing Aids

Arthur Schaub, Dipl. Phys.
Technology and Innovation Executive
Bernafon AG
Berne, Switzerland

Thieme
New York · Stuttgart

Thieme Medical Publishers, Inc.
333 Seventh Ave.
New York, NY 10001

Editor: Birgitta Brandenburg
Associate Editor: Ivy Ip
Vice President, Production and Electronic Publishing:
Anne T. Vinnicombe
Production Editor: Kenneth L. Chumbley, Publication
Services
Vice President, International Marketing and Sales:
Cornelia Schulze
Chief Financial Officer: Peter van Woerden
President: Brian D. Scanlan
Compositor: Aptara, Inc.
Printer: Everbest Printing Company, Ltd.

Important note: Medical knowledge is ever-changing. As new research and clinical experience broaden our knowledge, changes in treatment and drug therapy may be required. The authors and editors of the material herein have consulted sources believed to be reliable in their efforts to provide information that is complete and in accord with the standards accepted at the time of publication. However, in view of the possibility of human error by the authors, editors, or publisher of the work herein or changes in medical knowledge, neither the authors, editors, nor publisher, nor any other party who has been involved in the preparation of this work, warrants that the information contained herein is in every respect accurate or complete, and they are not responsible for any errors or omissions or for the results obtained from use of such information. Readers are encouraged to confirm the information contained herein with other sources. For example, readers are advised to check the product information sheet included in the package of each drug they plan to administer to be certain that the information contained in this publication is accurate and that changes have not been made in the recommended dose or in the contraindications for administration. This recommendation is of particular importance in connection with new or infrequently used drugs. Some of the product names, patents, and registered designs referred to in this book are in fact registered trademarks or proprietary names even though specific reference to this fact is not always made in the text. Therefore, the appearance of a name without designation as proprietary is not to be construed as a representation by the publisher that it is in the public domain.

Library of Congress Cataloging-in-Publication Data
Schaub, Arthur.
Digital hearing aids / Arthur Schaub.
p. ; cm.
Includes bibliographical references and index.
ISBN 978-1-60406-006-5 (alk. paper)
1. Hearing aids. 2. Signal processing—Digital
techniques. I. Title.
[DNLM: 1. Hearing Aids. 2. Amplifiers.
3. Analog-Digital Conversion. 4. Fourier Analysis.
WV 274 S313d 2008]
RF300.S318 2008
617.8'9—dc22
                                        2007051866

Printed in China
5 4 3 2 1
ISBN: 978-1-60406-006-5

This book is dedicated to Monika, my wife, and our daughters Julia and Linda—they always exercise patience when I am lost in thought, pondering some mathematical relationship.

Arthur Schaub
Bern, Switzerland

Contents

This is an amazing book. I have never read anything quite like it. The author has taken on the extraordinary challenge of bridging engineering and audiology. The author's basic training is in physics; he then specialized in electrical engineering. My own training is in audiology. With the advent of today's digital hearing aids, especially over the past 15 years, the paths of these normally very different fields have begun to intersect often.

The "collision" and communication between these two disciplines began in earnest when analog hearing aids in the mid-1990s began to incorporate wide dynamic range compression (WDRC) and multichannel technology. These attributes marked the pinnacle as well as the end of analog hearing aid technology. These WDRC hearing aids, for the most part, had two-channels and were programmable. Hearing aid technology had begun to "heat up" and increase on an exponential incline. Audiologists and other hearing health-care professionals were hard pressed to absorb, digest, and otherwise keep up with the burgeoning developments. Manufacturers began hiring audiologists to explain new technology. These same audiologists, however, had to pay daily visits to the engineers in the research and development corner of their companies to understand concepts they had never learned at university. The collision (and collusion) had begun.

In the late 1990s, the first digital hearing aids emerged. The pace of developments only got faster. Acoustic digital signal processing (DSP) continues to rack up further accomplishments in chip size reduction and processing speed. Today, it is "de rigueur" for hearing health-care professionals to be bombarded with additional features and benefits that are afforded by DSP. The context of features and benefits into the fitting of hearing aids is one thing; understanding how these work in a digital format is quite another. Hearing health-care professionals are trained more in the psychosocial realm, learning an interesting hybrid or fusion of anatomy, psychology, and basic electronics. We hear of bits and bytes, but we do not learn how DSP actually works. To be competent at what we do, audiologists and other hearing health care pro-

fessionals don't really *have* to learn in much detail how DSP works; otherwise most of us would not be working in our field. Further training in DSP is therefore quite optional. Hence, this book is not for everyone. It is, however, a wonderful entry for the audiologist or other hearing health care professional who is curious and wants to learn more. This book represents a valuable achievement by an engineer who develops DSP, to explain some of the rudiments of his knowledge base to hearing health care professionals who normally know quite little about this fascinating field.

Arthur Schaub writes in a straightforward manner. You will note that he uses relatively short sentences and refrains from flowery explanations and long-winded detail. Follow along and learn what he has to say. In the first part of the book (Chapters 1 to 4), he reviews the material with which most readers are quite familiar, such as, hearing aid styles, venting, etc. He also extends these topics, however, by exploring acoustic signal characteristics. In this manner, he lays a foundation for later chapters. He presents a preview of the main signal processing algorithms that many digital hearing aids utilize today as standard building blocks, such as WDRC, feedback cancellation, and adaptive or automatic program changes.

In the second part of his book (Chapters 5 to 10), he looks more closely at acoustic DSP in digital hearing aids. We gain new insights into how digital hearing aids actually work and what they achieve, as well as their limitations. At this point, we are still spared numerical digital signal representation. The focus here is on the concepts underlying the five essential functions of to digital hearing aids: amplification, acoustic directionality, noise reduction, feedback cancellation, and sound classification.

In the third part (Chapters 11 to 14), it is no longer possible to refrain from mathematical representation of DSP. The focus remains on essential concepts: the Fourier transform, digital FIR (finite impulse response) and IIR (infinite impulse response) filters, autocorrelation, and linear prediction. Here, however, the author deals with numerical explanations and refers often to Excel spreadsheet tables and simple formulas. He has prepared simple numerical examples to facilitate as precise a mental picture as possible. Although the examples are simple, they are still realistic – and probably challenging for most readers to follow. By the way, Arthur Schaub also told me that these chapters were the most challenging for him to write.

Here, a due diligence on the part of the reader will be rewarded in kind. These last few chapters must be read in the spirit in which they were written. Readers are encouraged to read in a mathematical language; for most, this will be the hardest part. To these readers especially, I encourage you to take the time to read the sections slowly. Look at the examples carefully and in detail, and see if you can follow the road where you are being led. When lost, relax, and try again later. Sometimes, a fresh start is all that is required. In summary, have patience here, and always realize that learning takes work. It usually takes years to reach a level of expertise in any field: mathematics, engineering, foreign languages, or playing chess. Acquiring the knowledge to obtain expertise is rather like a web. The challenge in learning consists in "linearizing" that web into a flow of thoughts. Follow the author's path in this book; you will emerge with a newfound appreciation for DSP in hearing aids.

Ted Venema, PhD
Coordinator
Hearing Instrument Specialist Program
School of Health Sciences
Community Services and Bio Technology
Connestoga College Institute of Technology
and Advanced Learning
Kitchener, Ontario, Canada

Preface

Since the mid-1990s, hearing aids have undergone a technological transformation. The instruments no longer process sound in an analog way, but digitally with an electronic processor.

Digital signal processing has led to innovations, for instance, new procedures to minimize the unwanted effects of acoustic feedback and background noise. Nevertheless, *digital signal processing* has also made it possible to enhance established procedures, for instance, the way to measure sound pressure level, or to realize wide dynamic range compression (WDRC). One such example is the ChannelFree technique from Bernafon AG (Berne, Switzerland).

Where can both practicing and prospective hearing-care professionals find basic information about digital hearing aid technology? How can they picture what is happening inside these instruments and what can they expect from the new technology? So far, the choice of textbooks dedicated to the subject has failed to keep up. Inspired by the management of Bernafon AG, this book goes some way to filling this gap. Containing numerous illustrations and example calculations, it concentrates on those topics essential for practicing and prospective hearing-care professionals.

The book is organized in three parts: Part I contains the basics and an overview, Part II presents a detailed analysis of state-of-the-art processing techniques, and Part III contains detailed technical information and numerical examples.

Chapter 1 explains a few basic physical concepts and provides an overview of acoustic signals: test signals from audiometry and signals from the acoustic environment – speech, music, and noise. We look at waveforms, spectra, and spectrograms.

Chapter 2 deals with hearing impairment; the discussion focuses on hearing loss, the loudness growth function, speech reception threshold, and word recognition, as well as the impact that hearing impairment has on hearing, understanding speech, and designing hearing aids.

Chapter 3 provides an overview of hearing aid characteristics. We look at customer satisfaction, hearing aid styles, and the impact of digital technology.

Chapter 4 deals with basic amplification schemes, starting from linear amplification, progressing to broadband compression and two-channel WDRC.

Chapters 5 and 6 talk about WDRC in digital hearing aids: their static behavior in Chapter 5 and their temporal behavior in Chapter 6. The static behavior describes how a hearing aid amplifies an unchanging, or slowly changing, input signal. This is related to how precisely different processing schemes match their amplification targets – the more precisely they do, the more flexibly the hearing aid can be fitted to an individual hearing loss. We consider three different approaches: WDRC using a transformation into the frequency domain, a filter bank, and a controllable filter.

The temporal behavior of WDRC, described in Chapter 6, investigates two aspects, how fast a processing scheme reacts to changes in the sound pressure level of the acoustic signal and the unwanted effects due to unfavorable temporal behavior. In the first part, we investigate the impact of using various methods for recording the sound pressure level of an acoustic signal. In considering the negative effects, we look at signal overshoot and loss in spectral contrast.

Chapters 7 to 10 present processing methods that only digital hearing aids can realize: adaptive directionality in Chapter 7, adaptive noise reduction in Chapter 8, adaptive feedback cancellation in Chapter 9, and sound classification in Chapter 10.

Chapter 11 shows how to process the acoustic signal in segments with the Fourier transform. Chapter 12 introduces digital filters. In Chapter 13, we look in detail at how to find the sound pressure level using digital signal processing. Chapter 14 presents the foundations of sound classification, autocorrelation and prediction. Finally, Chapter 15 recapitulates how everything fits together.

Acknowledgments

Looking back over the past 20 years, I can identify a key factor for success. One must have the capacity to look past immediate problems and everyday concerns and be motivated to tackle more distant goals. It is thanks to people with such foresight that I have had such interesting tasks to work on over the years. This, in turn, has led to this book, in the writing of which numerous colleagues have been generous with their assistance.

Special acknowledgments go to the manager of Bernafon AG, Erich Spahr, for commissioning me to write this book; my previous manager, Roland Küng, who had already initiated a collaboration with the ORL Clinic at the University Hospital of Zurich in the late 1980s; Prof. Dr. Norbert Dillier and Dr. Thomas Fröhlich, who carried out crucial preliminary work leading to the ChannelFree technique; Remo Leber for his collaboration on the Symbio and SwissEar hearing instruments: especially for his brilliant algorithm for feedback cancellation and his method for generating sample transfer functions for the controllable lattice filter; Jan Larsen, for encouraging me to implement the IC-design of the Symbio signal processing blocks using the hardware description language Verilog; Erich Zwyssig for preparing the entire Symbio IC to be ready for production; Monika Bertges Reber, who motivated me to investigate noise reduction; the previous manager of Bernafon AG, Peter Finnerup, for motivating Remo Leber and myself to tackle feedback cancellation and adaptive directionality; Simone Hänsli and Ursula Rytz, for assistance with stylistic elements; Anna Berg, Klaus-Dieter Butsch, and Thomas Trachsel, for painstakingly checking my manuscript, improving it with their many constructive suggestions; Sarah Bostock for translating the original German text into English; Neil Hockley for proofreading the English version—and finally, Ted Venema, author of *Compression for Clinicians*, and Mike Valente for their numerous suggestions to improve both the content and presentation.

Part I

Basics and Overview

1

Acoustic Signals

Our hearing lets us perceive the sounds around us; the sounds reach our ears as acoustic signals. Therefore, the sections in this first chapter deal with

1. *Basics*: anatomy of the ear, sound pressure and sound pressure level, graphical representations of acoustic signals (for a detailed discussion of the anatomy of the ear, see Møller, 2000, or Stach, 1998)
2. *Test signals in audiometry*: pure tones and band-limited noise
3. *Everyday acoustic signals*: speech, music, and noise

◆ Basics

Figure 1–1 shows a cross-section of the structure inside the human ear. The ear is made up of three main parts: the outer ear, the middle ear, and the inner ear.

The outer ear consists of the pinna and the external ear canal. Acoustic signals reach the outer ear as sound waves. The outer ear acts like a funnel, collecting these sounds and amplifying those parts of the signals that are especially important for our hearing.

The tympanic membrane forms an airtight barrier between the outer and middle ear. When sound waves hit the tympanic membrane, it begins to move about its equilibrium point in time with the sound pressure waves.

The middle ear contains three tiny bones, or ossicles, which are known as the malleus, incus, and stapes because of their shapes. They transmit and amplify the tympanic membrane's vibrations to the cochlea in the inner ear.

The inner ear consists on one side of the cochlea, and on the other side of the balance organ, which is not important for hearing. The cochlea transforms the mechanical vibrations into electrical nerve impulses that travel via the auditory nerve to the brain, where they form the actual impression of sound.

The human ear can perceive an enormous range of volume levels as **Fig. 1–2** shows. The physical measure for acoustic volume is sound pressure; its unit is the Pascal. The Pascal is named after the French philosopher, mathematician, and physicist Blaise Pascal, and is abbreviated to Pa.

The sound pressure of unbearably loud sound is a million times greater than the sound pressure of the quietest, just perceivable sound. The scale goes from 20 to 20,000,000 μPa. Here the abbreviation μPa is used for micro-Pascal – one millionth of a Pascal.

To avoid using such large numbers, sound pressure is usually converted into the more manageable sound pressure level (Everest, 2000; Kuttruff, 2000). As **Fig. 1–2** shows, this conversion results in a significantly smaller number range of 0 to 120 dB SPL. The abbreviation SPL stands for *sound pressure level*, and dB for *decibel*, a measure of logarithmic ratios named after the Scottish inventor Alexander Graham Bell.

For a sound pressure of p Pa, the sound pressure level L dB SPL is calculated as follows:

$$L = 10 \cdot \log_{10}(p^2/p_0^2)$$
$$= 20 \cdot \log_{10}(p/p_0) \qquad \text{(Eq. 1-1)}$$

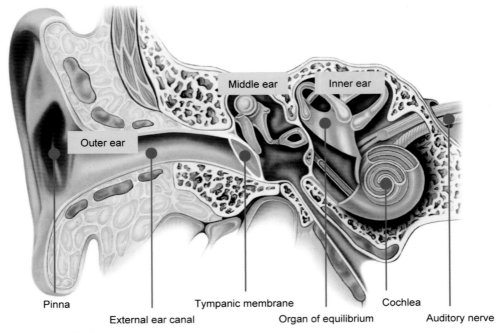

Middle ear

Inner ear

Outer ear

| Pinna | Tympanic membrane | Cochlea |
| External ear canal | Organ of equilibrium | Auditory nerve |

Figure 1–1   The human ear.

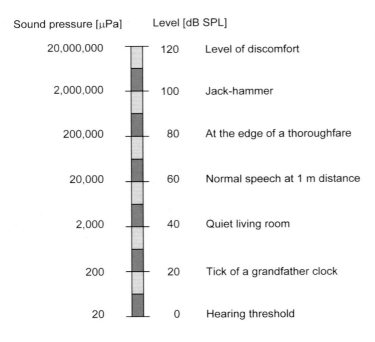

Sound pressure [µPa]   Level [dB SPL]

20,000,000	120	Level of discomfort
2,000,000	100	Jack-hammer
200,000	80	At the edge of a thoroughfare
20,000	60	Normal speech at 1 m distance
2,000	40	Quiet living room
200	20	Tick of a grandfather clock
20	0	Hearing threshold

Figure 1–2   Relationship between sound pressure and sound pressure level.

Table 1–1 Relationship between Changes in Sound Pressure and Sound Pressure Level

Sound Pressure	Sound Pressure Level
Twice as much	+6 dB
Half as much	−6 dB
Ten times as much	+20 dB
Ten times less	−20 dB

where p_0 denotes a reference pressure of 20 μPa.

Bel is the unit for the logarithmic ratio of squared sound pressure values; the factor 10 in the equation converts this value to the more usual and 10 times smaller unit *decibel*. And the factor 20 is instead used when the logarithm is calculated of the sound pressure ratio directly.

Figure 1–2 shows the relationship between sound pressure and sound pressure level graphically; therefore, it is unnecessary to go any deeper into the mathematics here. In addition, the figure shows the levels corresponding to typical hearing situations: 40 dB SPL represents a quiet living room, 60 dB SPL normal speech at a distance of one meter, etc.

If the sound pressure changes, then so does the value of the sound pressure level. **Table 1–1** shows the most important relationships.

In actual fact when the sound pressure doubles, it is not a change of exactly 6 dB, but rather $20 \cdot \log(2) = 6.03$ dB. It is usually sufficient, however, to use the rounded value of 6 in calculations.

Psychoacoustics uses the term *loudness* to describe how loud people subjectively perceive a specific sound. The next chapter will come back to this in more detail when we will look at the *loudness growth function*. For the moment it is enough to say that the loudness doubles when the sound level increases by 10 dB.

Before concluding this introductory section, we quickly take a look at the various graphical representations that will illustrate acoustic signals throughout the book:

◆ The *time domain graph* shows the waveform of sound pressure versus time. The first example in this book will illustrate pure tones in the Pure Tones subsection below. (**Figures 1-3a–1-3d.**)
◆ A *spectrum* shows the frequency content of an acoustic signal, exhibiting its low,

medium, and high frequency signal components; the levels of the different signal components are displayed along a frequency-axis. A first example will also appear in the Pure Tones subsection.

◆ The *spectrogram* (Baken & Orlikoff, 2000) uses frequency and time axes along with a color coding to represent the level of the acoustic signal at every point in time and frequency. The first example in this book will illustrate a speech signal in the Speech subsection.

◆ Test Signals in Audiometry

There are two types of signals to consider. In the first subsection, we will look at the signals used in pure-tone audiometry (Gelfand, 2001; Roeser et al, 2000); and the second subsection will present band-limited noise that is commonly used in *loudness scaling* (Brand and Hohmann, 2002; Kiessling et al, 1996).

Pure Tones

From a mathematical point of view, pure tones are sine waves. We will therefore quickly review the basic notions of amplitude, period, and frequency, and then look at the waveform and spectrum of different tones.

The term *period* refers to the repeat interval of a repetitive event; it is, therefore, a time, measured in seconds (abbreviation s). Acoustic signals usually involve smaller time intervals:

◆ Thousandths of seconds, known as milliseconds, abbreviated to ms
◆ Millionths of seconds, or microseconds, abbreviated to μs

The *frequency* of a signal describes how often an event repeats itself. The unit of frequency is the Hertz, named after the German physicist Heinrich Hertz, and is abbreviated to Hz. 1 Hz means 1 oscillation per second. Acoustic signals have frequencies in a range of around 20 Hz up to 20,000 Hz; 1,000 Hz is also known as 1 kilohertz – shortened to kHz.

Figures 1–3a—1–3d show the waveforms of four sinusoidal signals over a time interval of 10

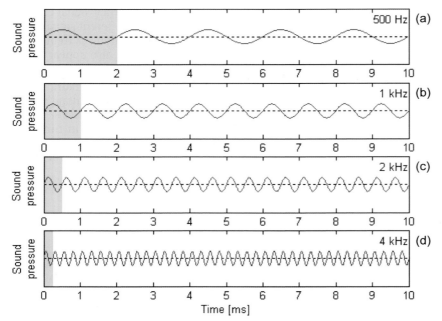

Figure 1–3   Pure tones with different frequencies: **(a)** 500 Hz, **(b)** 1 kHz, **(c)** 2 kHz, and **(d)** 4 kHz.

ms. All four tones display the same maximum sound pressure called the amplitude of the sinusoidal signal.

The first oscillation of each tone, in other words a single period, is marked in yellow. The periods of the sample tones are 2 ms, 1 ms, 500 μs, and 250 μs, and their frequencies – the inverse of the period – are 500 Hz, 1 kHz, 2 kHz, and 4 kHz, respectively.

The term *octave* is used to describe a frequency interval whose highest frequency is twice as large as its lowest. Therefore, in the sequence of the four sample tones, each tone lays 1 octave from the next.

If all four sample tones were generated at the same time, then the resulting signal would have a sound pressure equal to the sum of all four tones combined. **Figure 1–4a** shows this compound signal. From the waveform it is scarcely possible to see the four separate tones, which make up the signal. The spectrum in **Fig. 1–4b** shows this much better. This graph shows a spectral line of 75 dB amplitude at each of the four signal frequencies. This consistency in level is a result of the fact that the initial tones were generated with the same amplitude.

In spectrum diagrams it is usual to make the frequency-axis logarithmic. In this way the four frequencies, which lie at one-octave intervals, appear with equal spacing.

Before concluding this subsection, let us verify the relationship between sound pressure and sound pressure level as displayed in **Table 1–1**. **Figures 1–5a–1–5c** show the waveforms of a 1 kHz tone with different amplitudes, and **Figs. 1–5d** to **1–5f** show the spectra.

The amplitude in **Fig. 1–5b** is 10 times that in **Fig. 1–5a**. The level increases accordingly by 20 dB from 55 dB to 75 dB. From **Fig. 1–5b** to **Fig. 1–5c** the amplitude doubles, resulting in an increase in level of 6 dB from 75 dB to 81 dB.

Band-limited Noise

In audiometry, noise signals are often limited to a frequency band one third of an octave wide (International Electrotechnical Commission [IEC], 1985; Möser, 2004). There are 18 of these third octave bands in the frequency range between 160 Hz and 8 kHz. Later on in this subsection, we will look at two examples of noise signals limited to one-third octave bands.

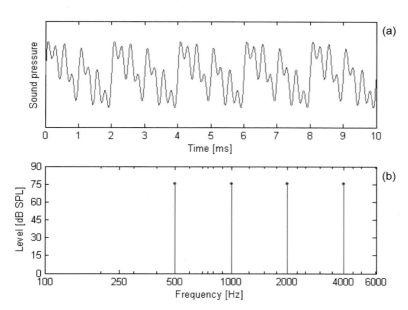

Figure 1–4 A compound signal: **(a)** waveform and **(b)** spectrum.

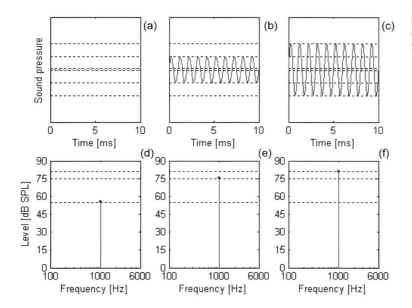

Figure 1–5 1 kHz tone with different amplitudes: **(a–c)** waveforms and **(d–f)** spectra.

First, however, the focus is on *white noise*, which serves as a starting point to derive band-limited noise signals. White noise gets its name from light. Light appears to be white when all colors (i.e., the different frequencies) are equally present. Similarly, signal compo-nents at all frequencies are equally present in white noise.

Figure 1–6a shows the waveform of a white noise signal. The shape of the waveform is ran-dom, in contrast to that of pure tones. **Figure 1–6b** shows the spectrum: the sound levels of all

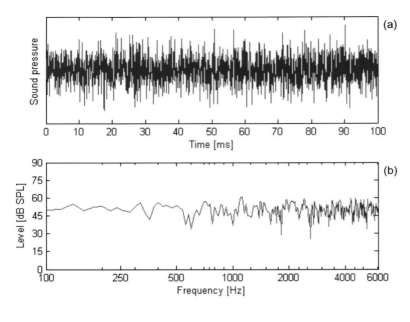

Figure 1–6   White noise: **(a)** wave-form and **(b)** spectrum.

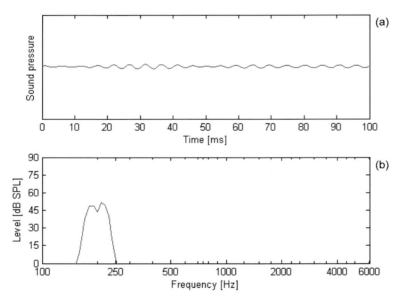

Figure 1–7   Third octave band noise at 200 Hz: **(a)** waveform and **(b)** spectrum.

signal components are equal over the entire frequency range from 100 Hz to 6 kHz, apart from small instantaneous random differences.

Filtering white noise with a band-pass filter produces band-limited noise. **Figure 1–7a** shows the waveform of a noise signal limited to a third octave band at 200 Hz. **Figure 1–7b** shows the signal's spectrum and confirms that it is band-limited.

As with a 200 Hz tone, there are 20 oscillations during the 100-ms time interval in **Fig. 1–7a**. However, in contrast to a pure tone, the amplitude also varies, which is typical behavior when signal components within a narrow fre-

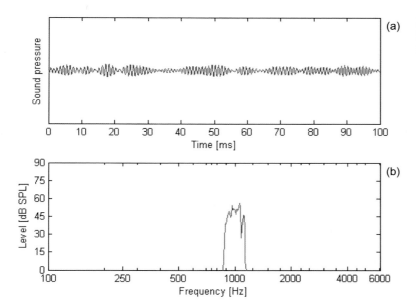

(a)

(b)

Figure 1–8 Third octave band noise at 1 kHz: **(a)** waveform and **(b)** spectrum.

quency range interact. This is similar to the beating that two pure tones of almost the same frequency produce.

Figure 1–8 shows a further example: a noise signal limited to a third octave band at 1 kHz. In this example, it is even easier to see that the amplitude oscillates in an irregular manner. Both the waveform in **Fig. 1–8a** and the spectrum in **Fig. 1–8b** shows the different frequency content with respect to the previous example.

◆ Everyday Acoustic Signals

The theme of this section comprises the acoustic signals that surround us in everyday life. They break down into three categories, which we will look at one by one: speech, music, and noise.

Speech

Speech enables us to communicate with one another in a highly efficient way. For this reason, it is the most important acoustic signal of all for us. Speech consists of a sequence of sounds, or phonemes, which differ greatly from one another in both time and frequency characteristics. This section will present the phonemes in a single

word; for a thorough discussion see Ladefoged (2001), Cassidy and Harrington (1999), Stevens (1998), or Coleman et al (1993), for example.

We will look in detail at the word "understand," in particular:

◆ The waveform in **Fig. 1–9a**

◆ The spectrogram in **Fig. 1–9b**

◆ The waveform of each individual phoneme in **Figs. 1–10a—1–10i**

◆ The spectra of single phonemes in **Figs. 1–11a—1–11d**

Figure 1–9a shows the different phonemes, following one after the other to make up the word "understand"; they can be distinguished by the differences in sound pressure. The different letters are shown alongside the signal, showing which phoneme each signal section consists of. It is amazing how the phonemes vary in duration, and the long pause – over 50 ms – before the stop /t/ is amazing too.

The spectrogram in **Fig. 1–9b** shows the structure of the signal, by breaking it down into time and frequency components. Time runs along the x-axis, as with the standard time domain graph in **Fig. 1–9a.** The y-axis, however, shows the frequency rather than amplitude, over a range of 0 to 6 kHz. The different colors indicate increasing levels from −25 dB up to +75 dB SPL – in the order blue, green, yellow,

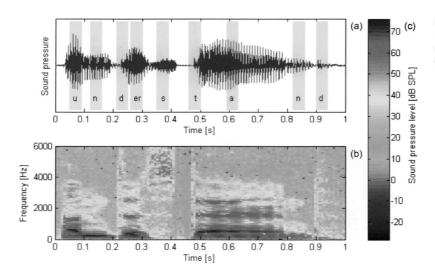

Figure 1–9 The word "understand": **(a)** waveform, **(b)** spectrogram, and **(c)** color code.

orange, red, and finally brown, as shown in **Fig. 1–9c**. This scale is used for all further spectrograms in this chapter.

A few features of the spectrogram in **Fig. 1–9b** are particularly striking:

◆ The sibilant /s/ is predominately made up of high frequency components.

◆ The stops /t/ and /d/ are short in duration, but are made up of a large range of frequency components from very low to very high.

◆ Low frequency components dominate in the vowel sounds, /u/, /er/, and /æ/, as well as the nasal sound /n/. In addition local maxima can be seen, called *formants*, which allow us to distinguish between the different vowels.

Figures 1–10a—1–10i show the waveforms of those segments, which are marked yellow in **Fig. 1–9a**. The larger scale on the time axis enables us to discern certain features:

◆ In voiced sounds the vocal folds inside the larynx cause periodic peaks in the signal. Examples are the vowels /u/, /er/, and /æ/ in **Figs. 1–10a, 1–10d, and 1–10g**, as well as the nasal sound /n/ in **Figs. 1–10b** *and* **1–10h**. In **Fig. 1–10a** the signal peaks occur at around 53, 61, 69, 78, and 86 ms.

The signal decays between each of these successive peaks, according to the shape of the resonant system – our vocal tract, which includes our throat, mouth, tongue, and lips. We rapidly form our whole resonating vocal tract in a different way for each phoneme.

The peaks become more noticeable as the mouth is opened wider when speaking a vowel sound. In contrast, the peaks in **Fig. 1–10b**, showing the nasal sound /n/, have largely fallen away because most of the signal leaves via the nose instead of the mouth.

◆ In unvoiced phonemes the sound pressure generated is irregular. Examples of this are the sibilant /s/ in **Fig. 1–10e** and the stop /t/ in **Fig. 1–10f**.

The /s/ sound consists of noise, caused by a continuous flow of air, which generates turbulence between the top and bottom rows of teeth.

The stop /t/ is distinctive because of both its preceding pause and its short duration. The pause occurs when the tip of the tongue presses against the teeth-ridge forming a seal. A stop sound is short in duration because we release the seal abruptly, once an increased air pressure has built up behind it. In the case of other stops the seal can be created in various ways, for example with

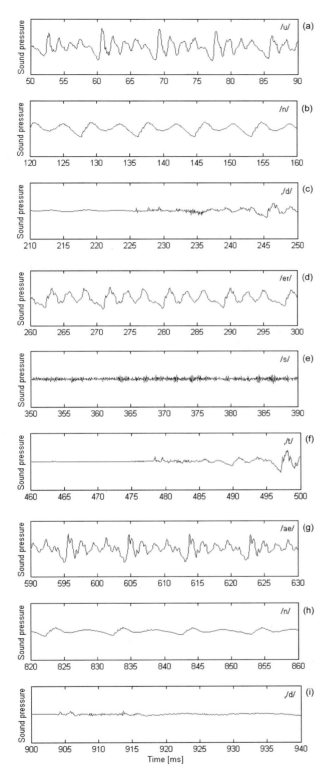

Figure 1–10   The phonemes of the word "understand" : **(a)** /u/, **(b)** /n/, **(c)** /d/, **(d)** /er/, **(e)** /s/, **(f)** /t/, **(g)** /æ/, **(h)** /n/, and **(i)** /d/.

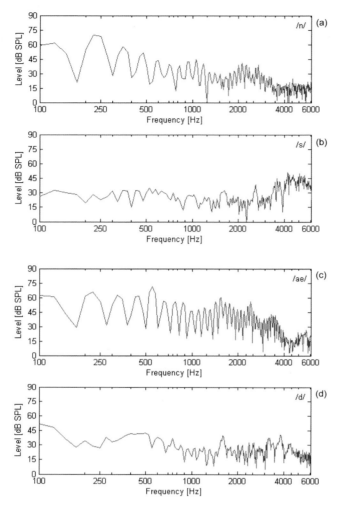

Figure 1–11   Spectra of various phonemes of the word "understand": **(a)** /n/, **(b)** /s/, **(c)** /æ/, and **(d)** /d/.

the lips in the case of /p/ and /b/. Within a word the stops last around 10 ms and are followed on by a vowel in this example. At the end of the word "understand" we see that the stop /d/ lasts for somewhat longer.

Figures 1–11a—1–11d show the spectra of the phonemes /n/, /s/, /æ/, and /d/. Comparing these graphs with the spectrogram in **Fig. 1–9b** confirms the correspondence between level and color coding. In addition the diagrams reveal the following features:

◆ In voiced phonemes the spectrum contains regular peaks.

   Example: the nasal /n/ in **Fig. 1–11a** and the vowel /æ/ in **Fig. 1–11c**.

The waveform of the nasal phoneme /n/ in **Fig. 1–10b** exhibits a period slightly greater than 8 ms. This corresponds to a frequency of around 120 Hz. In **Fig. 1–11a** we see the first peak in the spectrum at just over 100 Hz, and further peaks occur at each multiple of 120 Hz, which is at 240 Hz, 360 Hz, etc.

◆ In unvoiced phonemes the spectrum shows irregular behavior.

   Example: the sibilant /s/ in **Fig. 1–11b** and the stop /d/ in **Fig. 1–11d**.

The spectrum of the sibilant /s/ clearly increases in the higher frequencies from 2 kHz upwards.

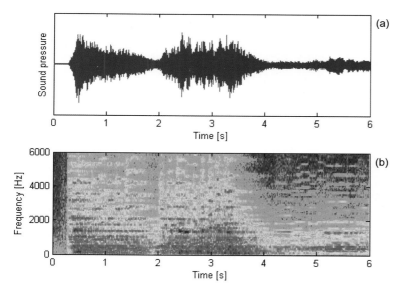

Figure 1–12 An example of classical music: **(a)** waveform and **(b)** spectrogram.

In contrast the spectrum of the stop /d/ is mostly flat, only increasing in the low frequencies from around 250 Hz downwards.

Music

Music speaks to us in a way almost nothing else does, and can even influence our mood. It lies outside the scope of this book to discuss all of the vast number of different musical styles that exist; we will instead look at just two examples:

◆ Classical music: a symphony orchestra
◆ Easy listening music: flute and guitar

Waveforms and spectrograms will illustrate 6-s-long time segments of both examples. Finally, we will look in more detail at the flute and guitar sample, in particular at the waveform and spectrum of a much shorter 40 ms extract.

Figure 1–12a shows the opening bars of one movement in a Beethoven symphony. During the first 4 s both string and wind instruments are playing, whereas in the remaining 2 s the wind instruments are playing alone. The participation of changing numbers of instruments leads to differing sound pressures.

Figure 1–12b shows the spectrogram of the same sample. The signal components reach far higher frequencies at the start, when both types of instruments are playing. Toward the end, when the strings have stopped, and only the wind instruments remain, the high frequency components have almost disappeared.

Figure 1–13a shows the waveform for another 6-s-long sample, this time from a piece of music written for flute and guitar. In this example the sound pressure remains within a more or less constant range for the entire duration. **Figure 1–13b** shows the corresponding spectrogram.

The spectrograms in **Fig. 1–12b** and **Fig. 1–13b** both reveal distinctive features that are typical of music:

◆ Signal components, which are typically spread over a large range of frequencies: from close to 0 Hz up to, and well in excess of, the 6 kHz displayed here
◆ Countless local minimum and maximum values along the frequency axis: the tone, consisting of a fundamental, or base tone, and harmonics, which occur at multiples of the fundamental
◆ Frequent and abrupt changes in the tonal pattern along the time axis: the rhythm, especially apparent in the spectrogram of **Fig. 1–13b**

Figure 1–14a shows a short signal extract of the flute and guitar piece. There are around $19\frac{1}{2}$ oscillations in the 40-ms segment—equivalent to a fundamental frequency of around 490 Hz. The spectrum in **Fig. 1–14b** shows a corresponding peak at just under

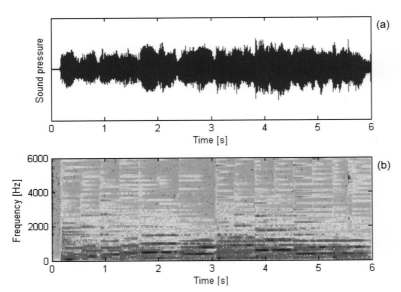

(a)

(b)

Figure 1–13 An example of easy listening music: **(a)** waveform and **(b)** spectrogram.

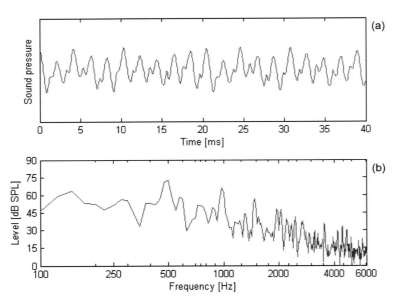

(a)

(b)

Figure 1–14 A short segment of easy listening music: **(a)** waveform and **(b)** spectrum.

500 Hz, as well as further peaks at multiples of the fundamental: 1 kHz, 1.5 kHz, etc.

Noise

The diversity of background noises is enormous: a babbling stream, raindrops drumming on the window, leaves rustling in the wind, a dog barking, church bells chiming, the telephone ringing, etc. Conveying a thorough overview of all these signals exceeds the scope of this book, so once again we will look at just two examples:

◆ A monotonous noise: a train traveling through a tunnel

◆ A pulsed noise: the clattering sound made by doing the dishes

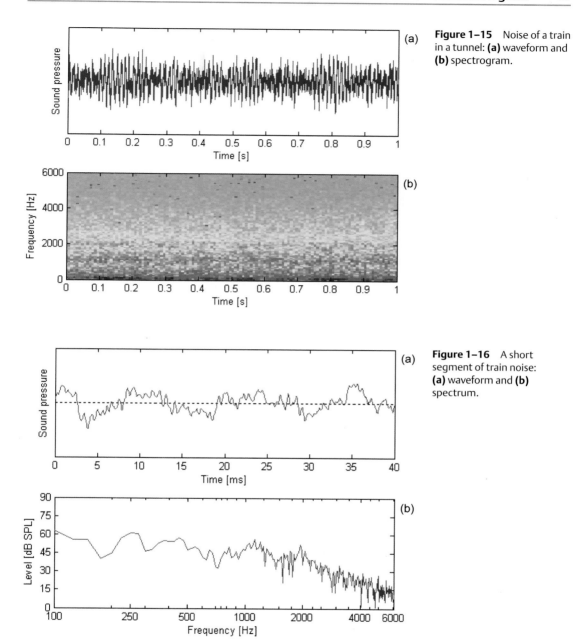

Figure 1–15 Noise of a train in a tunnel: **(a)** waveform and **(b)** spectrogram.

Figure 1–16 A short segment of train noise: **(a)** waveform and **(b)** spectrum.

Waveforms and spectrograms will illustrate 1-s-long samples of both signals. Then we will look at waveforms and spectra of shorter 40-ms samples.

Figure 1–15a displays the waveform of the noise made by a train traveling through a tunnel. Over the entire 1-s time interval the sound

pressure remains within a more or less constant range. The spectrogram in **Fig. 1–15b** shows that low frequency components dominate the signal, and that the level falls off monotonically toward higher frequencies.

Figure 1–16a shows the sound pressure of a shorter, 40-ms segment of the same sound

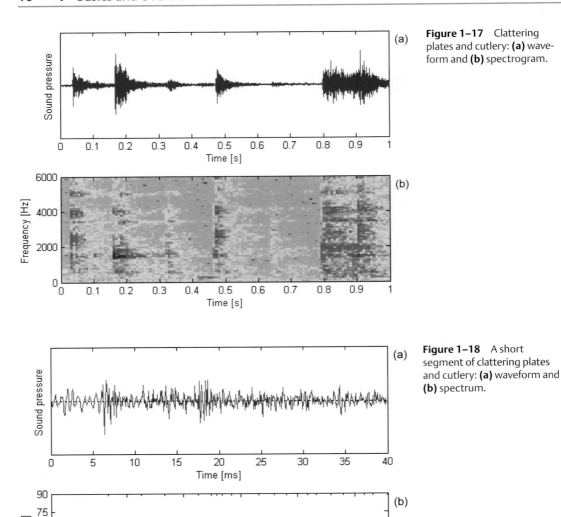

Figure 1–17   Clattering plates and cutlery: **(a)** waveform and **(b)** spectrogram.

Figure 1–18   A short segment of clattering plates and cutlery: **(a)** waveform and **(b)** spectrum.

sample. Subsequent intersections of the marked zero line generally lie more than 1 ms apart. This indicates that the signal's dominant components lie below 500 Hz. The spectrum in **Fig. 1–16b** confirms this finding. The spectrum decreases from the low to the high frequencies, with random minima and maxima occurring in between.

Figure 1–17a shows the waveform of an acoustic signal generated by clattering plates and cutlery together. The waveform exhibits considerable modulation, i.e., its sound pressure repeatedly increases and decreases. The spectrogram in **Fig. 1–17b** lets us see the modulation as well. And it also shows that signal components over the entire frequency range contribute to the noise signal—from close to 0 Hz to and exceeding 6 kHz.

Figure 1–18a shows a short 40-ms extract of the noise signal generated by clattering plates and cutlery. In this case, the signal passes through the zero line much more frequently.

The spectrum in **Fig. 1–18b** exhibits a peak just below 1.5 kHz. In **Fig. 1–18a**, there are $7^1/_2$ oscillations during the first 5 ms – equivalent to the peak at 1.5 kHz in the spectrum.

◆ Summary

In this chapter, we first looked at some basic aspects of our sense of hearing. The subsequent sections presented audiometric test signals and signals from everyday life. The analysis illustrated these signals by means of three graphical representations: a time domain graph shows the waveform of a signal, a spectrum depicts the frequency content of a signal, and a spectrogram uses a color code to represent the level of each signal component at every point in time and frequency.

References

Baken, R.J., and Orlikoff, R.F. (2000). Clinical measurement of speech and voice. Clifton Park, NY: Thomson Delmar Learning.

Brand, T., and Hohmann, V. (2002). An adaptive procedure for categorical loudness scaling, Journal of the Acoustical Society of America, 112(4), 1597–1604.

Cassidy, S., and Harrington, J. (1999). Techniques in speech acoustics. New York/Heidelberg/Berlin: Springer.

Coleman, J.S., Greenwood, A., and Olive, J.P. (1993). Acoustics of American English speech: A dynamic approach. New York/Heidelberg/Berlin: Springer.

Everest, F.A. (2000). Master handbook of acoustics (4th ed.). New York: McGraw-Hill.

Gelfand, S.A. (2001). Essentials of audiology. New York: Thieme Medical Publishers.

International Electrotechnical Commission. (1985). IEC 60268-1. Sound system equipment, part 1: General (2nd ed.). Geneva: International Electrotechnical Commission.

Kiessling, J., Schubert, M., and Archut, A. (1996). Adaptive fitting of hearing instruments by category loudness scaling (ScalAdapt), Scandinavian Audiology, 25(3), 153–160.

Kuttruff, H. (2000). Room acoustics. London: Spon Press.

Ladefoged P. (2001). Vowels and consonants: An introduction to the sounds of languages. Oxford: Blackwell Publishing.

Møller, A.R. (2000). Hearing: Its physiology and pathophysiology. Amsterdam: Elsevier.

Möser, M. (2004). Engineering acoustics: An introduction to noise control. New York/Heidelberg/Berlin: Springer.

Roeser, R.J., Valente, M., and Hosford-Dunn, H. (2000). Audiology: Diagnosis. New York: Thieme Medical Publishers.

Stach B.A. (1998). Clinical Audiology: An introduction. Clifton Park, NY: Thomson Delmar Learning.

Stevens, K.N. (1998). Acoustic phonetics. Cambridge, MA: MIT Press.

2

Hearing Impairment

This chapter consists of four sections that deal with

1. *Hearing loss*: the difference between a hearing-impaired person's hearing threshold and that of listeners with normal hearing
2. The *loudness growth function*: a subjective measure of how well people perceive acoustic signals with sound pressure levels above their hearing threshold
3. *Speech reception threshold* and *word recognition*: tests that are useful to assess hearing and that aid in the selection and fitting of hearing aids
4. The *impact of a hearing impairment*: on hearing, understanding speech, and designing hearing aids

These audiological concepts comprise an enormous amount of information. The following sections, however, provide only a brief review – for more details see Stach (1998), Gelfand (2001), Sataloff and Sataloff (1993), Roeser et al (2000), or Katz (2001).

◆ Hearing Loss

A person first notices a hearing loss when the *hearing thresholds* increase. The hearing threshold is the minimum sound pressure level required to perceive a pure tone. A person with a hearing loss needs a higher sound pressure level, and so has a higher threshold, than a person with normal hearing. The *difference* between this increased threshold and the threshold of normal hearing listeners is the *hearing loss*; it is commonly expressed in dB HL, where HL stands for hearing level.

Pure-tone audiometry (Gelfand, 2001; Roeser et al, 2000) uses sinusoidal test signals, thereby making it possible to determine the hearing threshold separately at different frequencies. There are nine standard audiometric measurement frequencies: 250 Hz, 500 Hz, 1 kHz, 1.5 kHz, 2 kHz, 3 kHz, 4 kHz, 6 kHz, and 8 kHz.

The curve in **Fig. 2–1** indicates the hearing thresholds for listeners with normal hearing (American National Standards Institute [ANSI], 1996), over a frequency range from 250 Hz to 8 kHz. The values hold for pure tones presented via an earphone to one ear only.

The hearing loss of a hearing-impaired person is determined by calculating the *difference* between the individual hearing thresholds and the values of the curve in **Fig. 2–1** for each measurement frequency. It is common practice to enter the results in a diagram called an *audiogram*. We will shortly turn our attention to four sample audiograms, but first we will look at three notions that further characterize hearing loss:

1. *Type*: relates to where a disorder causes hearing impairment – all along the path from the outer ear to the auditory centers in the brain
2. *Degree*: refers to the severity of hearing loss – usually to the *pure-tone-average* (i.e., the average of pure-tone thresholds at 500 Hz, 1 kHz, and 2 kHz) these frequencies are also known as the *speech frequencies*

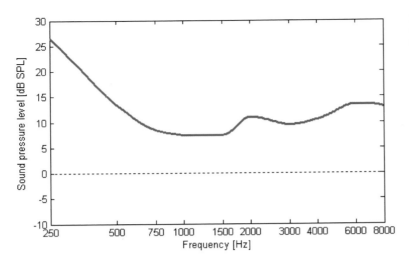

Figure 2-1 The hearing threshold of normal hearing listeners.

3. *Configuration*: comprises the *shape* of a hearing loss when displayed in an *audiogram*, but also a few more characteristics

Type

There are four different types of hearing loss: *conductive*, *sensorineural*, *mixed*, and *central*.

1. A *conductive* hearing loss is caused by a disorder in either the outer or middle ear, such that the sound is no longer conducted efficiently to the inner ear. This is like having an earplug in the ear: soft sounds are no longer audible and intense sounds are reduced in loudness.

   Medical treatment or surgery can often correct this disorder. If not, amplifying the acoustic signal usually produces good results. *Conductive* hearing losses account for up to 10% of all hearing losses.

   Common causes are cerumen buildup, infection of the ear canal or middle ear, fluid in the middle ear, perforated tympanic membrane, dislocation or fixation of the ossicles in the middle ear, tumors, and others.

2. A *sensorineural* hearing loss occurs when the cochlea (*sensory*) in the inner ear is affected – and possibly also the auditory nerve (*neural*). This changes the way a person perceives loudness: soft sounds again become inaudible, but intense sounds are heard as loudly as by listeners who have

normal hearing – in fact, the "floor" of their hearing sensitivity has raised while the "ceiling" of their loudness discomfort has remained the same.

There is currently no method to correct sensorineural disorder by medical treatment or surgery. Amplifying the acoustic signal helps but cannot return hearing to normal; it usually makes sense to apply more gain to soft sounds and less gain to loud sounds, thus compensating for the altered loudness perceptions. Sensorineural hearing losses account for the vast majority of all losses; estimates range up to 90%.

Common causes are aging, loud noise, viral infections, medication, injury, genetics, tumors, and others.

3. A *mixed* hearing loss includes both *conductive and sensorineural* components. In other words, there is damage to the outer or middle ear and also to the cochlea in the inner ear or to the auditory nerve or both.

4. A *central* hearing loss is caused by a disorder in the central auditory nervous system. This usually leaves pure-tone thresholds close to normal, but manifests itself in poor word recognition scores and speech reception thresholds. We will briefly look at these tests in the Speech Reception Threshold and Word Recognition section.

There is currently no treatment available for *central* hearing loss. *Central* hearing losses are rare. Common causes are tumors,

Table 2–1 Degree of Hearing Loss

Degree of Loss	Range in dB HL
Normal	−10 to 10
Minimal	10 to 25
Mild	25 to 40
Moderate	40 to 55
Moderately severe	55 to 70
Severe	70 to 90
Profound	>90

Source: Data from Stach, B. A. (1998). Clinical audiology: An introduction. Clifton Park, NY: Thomson Delmar Learning. Adapted by permission.

Table 2–2 Shape of Hearing Loss

Shape of Loss	Characteristic
Flat	Thresholds are within 20 dB of each other across the frequency range
Rising	Thresholds for low frequencies are at least 20 dB poorer than for high frequencies
Sloping	Thresholds for high frequencies are at least 20 dB poorer than for low frequencies
Low-frequency	Hearing loss is restricted to the low-frequency region of the audiogram
High-frequency	Hearing loss is restricted to the high-frequency region of the audiogram
Precipitous	Steeply sloping high frequency hearing loss of at least 20 dB per octave

Source: Data from Stach, B. A. (1998). Clinical audiology: An introduction. Clifton Park, NY: Thomson Delmar Learning. Adapted by permission.

a lesion caused by stroke, or other changes in neural structure.

Degree

Table 2–1 classifies hearing thresholds into seven categories. The first two categories relate to normal hearing and minimal loss, respectively. Minimal loss infers no significant difficulty in the ability to hear and understand speech. So, there remain five categories that indicate varying severity of hearing loss: *mild*, *moderate*, *moderately severe*, *severe*, and *profound*.

The degree of hearing loss usually refers to the *pure-tone average* (i.e., the average of the thresholds at the *speech frequencies* 500 Hz, 1 kHz, and 2 kHz). But it is also possible to use the terms for the thresholds at other frequencies, when explicitly stating so.

Configuration

One aspect of *configuration* relates to the *shape* of hearing loss (i.e., the amount of loss across frequencies). **Table 2–2** defines six different shapes: *flat*, *rising*, *sloping*, *low-frequency*, *high-frequency*, and *precipitous*. We will shortly turn to different *shapes* when looking at the sample *audiograms* in **Fig. 2–2**.

Audiograms follow some conventions in displaying hearing loss. The x-axis shows the frequency on a logarithmic scale, and the y-axis shows the hearing loss in dB HL. In an unusual way, the hearing loss scale has its lowest value at the top of the y-axis, and increases in value toward the bottom.

This section started with the definition of hearing loss: the hearing threshold of a hear-

ing-impaired person minus that of listeners with normal hearing. As a result, the 0-dB line in the audiogram corresponds to the continuous threshold curve in **Fig. 2–1**.

The hearing losses in the sample audiograms differ from one another in both *shape* and *degree*:

- **Figure 2–2a**
  - Shape: sloping. The thresholds at high frequencies exceed those at low frequencies by more than 20 dB.
  - Degree: mild. Pure-tone average $= {}^1\!/_3 \cdot (25 + 40 + 45)$ dB $\cong 37$ dB

- **Figure 2–2b**
  - Shape: flat. The thresholds across frequencies are all within 20 dB from each other.
  - Degree: moderate. Pure-tone average $= {}^1\!/_3 \cdot (45 + 50 + 55)$ dB $= 50$ dB

- **Figure 2–2c**
  - Shape: rising. The thresholds at the low frequencies exceed those at the high frequencies by more than 20 dB.
  - Degree: moderately severe. Pure-tone average $= {}^1\!/_3 \cdot (75 + 60 + 50) \cong 62$ dB

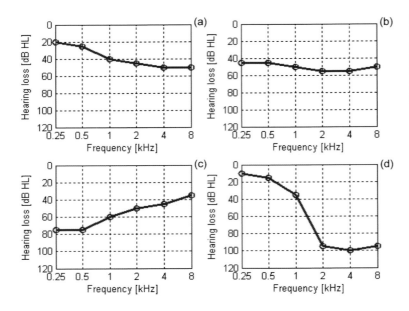

Figure 2–2 Examples of hearing loss: **(a)** mild sloping hearing loss, **(b)** moderate flat hearing loss, **(c)** moderately severe, rising hearing loss, and **(d)** precipitous hearing loss, profound at 2 kHz and above.

◆ **Figure 2–2d**

  ◆ Shape: precipitous. Slope exceeds 20 dB within the octave from 1kHz to 2 kHz.

  ◆ Degree: profound at 2 kHz and higher frequencies – above 90 dB

The *configuration* of hearing loss covers more than *shape*; the additional aspects raise the following questions:

Bilateral versus *unilateral*: Does a hearing loss affect both ears or only one?

Symmetrical versus *asymmetrical*: Does a hearing loss show the same *degree* and *shape* in both ears or are they different?

Stable versus *fluctuating*: Does a hearing loss remain the same over time or does it change, i.e., get better at times and then worse again?

Progressive versus *sudden*: Has a hearing loss evolved over years or occurred rapidly?

Hearing loss captures the thresholds of hearing, but disregards what happens above thresholds. Another procedure measures hearing above thresholds: *loudness scaling*. And its results establish the *loudness growth function*, the subject of the next section.

◆ Loudness Growth Function

Loudness scaling (Kiessling et al, 1996; Brand & Hohmann, 2002) allows us to measure the *loudness growth function* at each of the audiometric frequencies. The test signal is usually band-limited noise, limited to standard third octave bands (International Electrotechnical Commission, 1985).

The subjective loudness of a sound gives the *loudness growth function*. This subjective loudness is gauged by asking a person to classify the sound pressure level according to a list of categories, for instance:

1. Very soft
2. Soft
3. Comfortable, but slightly soft
4. Comfortable
5. Comfortable, but slightly loud
6. Loud, but OK
7. Uncomfortably loud

Often, when carrying out *loudness scaling* by using a computer, input devices allow a finer classification into up to fifty categories. However, if the measurement results are shown graphically, normally fewer categories are used, for instance only five as with the examples in this section:

1. Very soft
2. Soft
3. Medium
4. Loud
5. Very loud

Figure 2–3 shows the loudness growth function of a hearing-impaired person (red) against that of listeners with normal hearing (blue) at a measurement frequency of 2 kHz. The red circles show measurement points, from which a mathematical procedure calculates the continuous loudness growth function. The green lines indicate how much more sound pressure level the hearing-impaired person needs to perceive the same impression of loudness as a normal hearing person. To that end, soft sounds typically need more amplification than loud sounds, in this example around 30 dB versus only 6 dB.

The abnormal growth of loudness is typical for *sensorineural* hearing loss and the technical term is *recruitment*. For the hearing-impaired person soft sounds are inaudible; intense sounds, however, are at least as loud

as a listener with normal hearing perceives them. This is a well-known effect: hearing-impaired persons often do not understand soft speech, but complain that loud speech is too loud.

Just as the hearing loss is different in value at different frequencies, so the *loudness growth function* generally differs at each frequency. **Figure 2–4** shows the results of measurements at 500 Hz, 1 kHz, 2 kHz, and 4 kHz; each of the four diagrams depicts the *loudness growth function* of a hearing-impaired person alongside that of listeners with normal hearing:

◆ **Figure 2–4a:** At 500 Hz the hearing-impaired person's loudness growth function is close to normal.

◆ **Figure 2–4b:** At 1 kHz the hearing-impaired person's loudness growth function starts off at 25 dB HL for very soft sounds, but gradually approaches the values of normal hearing as the sound pressure level rises to 90 dB HL.

◆ **Figure 2–4c:** At 2 kHz the hearing-impaired person's loudness growth function begins at 40 dB HL, then increases more steeply than that of normal hearing persons, and again gradually approaches normal values at high sound pressure levels.

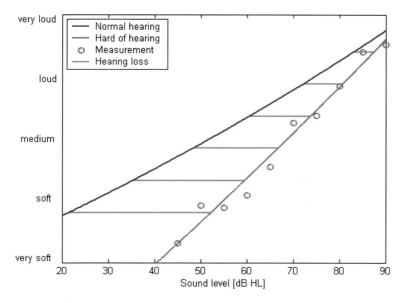

Figure 2–3 Example of a loudness growth function.

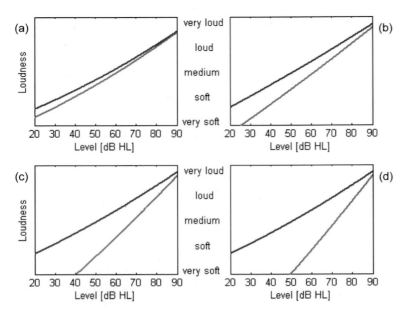

Figure 2–4   Loudness growth functions at different frequencies: **(a)** at 500 Hz, **(b)** at 1 kHz, **(c)** at 2 kHz, and **(d)** at 4 kHz.

◆ **Figure 2–4d:** At 4 kHz the hearing-impaired person's loudness growth function sets off at 50 dB HL, increases even more steeply and again approaches the values of normal hearing as the level increases.

Loudness scaling has not found widespread use; for a discussion on pros and cons, see Dillon (2001). Some researchers even claim that threshold data are sufficient to predict hearing above threshold – see Elberling (1999).

◆ **Speech Reception Threshold and Word Recognition**

Testing for *speech reception threshold* and *word recognition* is a part of *speech audiometry*. As the name implies, these procedures use speech signals as test stimulus.

The *speech reception threshold* is the lowest level at which a person can hear and correctly repeat 50% of the test words presented to him or her. The test usually presents two-syllabic words with equal emphasis on both syllables, usually called *spondaic words*; examples are "baseball," "railroad," or "hotdog."

Word recognition tests evaluate how well a person can hear and correctly repeat test words commonly presented at a comfortable loudness level. The test signal in this case usually consists of single-syllabic words, and the percentage of correctly recognized words determines the test result.

Speech as a test stimulus involves all parts of the auditory system, from the outer ear to complex nervous processes in the brain. Sinusoidal signals and band-limited noise, however, imply simpler tasks to the auditory brain centers. *Speech audiometry* thus complements the audiologist's diagnosis.

Likewise, *speech audiometry* comes closer to what hearing is about in everyday life. This holds even more for some further tests that address hearing in noise, such as HINT (Nilsson et al, 1994) or the SIN test (Kalikow et al, 1977). The more realistic the tests are, the more effective they are in evaluating the benefits of hearing aid use.

◆ **Impact of a Hearing Impairment**

Next, we will look at what a hearing impairment means for hearing and understanding speech. And then we will consider its influence on hearing aid design.

Impact of a Hearing Impairment on Hearing and Understanding Speech

Table 2–3 summarizes how hearing loss of different degree impacts on communication. The effect ranges from having difficulty in hearing faint speech to not hearing loud sounds at all.

Figure 2–5 illustrates two examples: the sloping hearing loss and the precipitous hearing loss described in the Hearing Loss section. The diagram shows different sounds, laid out according to their frequencies and sound pressure levels. Normal hearing listeners perceive all of the sounds – including all the speech phonemes in the pink shaded area, outlined in red.

Hearing-impaired persons, however, only hear sounds at sound pressure levels above their hearing threshold (i.e., the sounds in **Fig. 2–5**

Table 2–3   Impact of Hearing Loss on Communication

Degree of Loss	Effect on Communication
Minimal	Difficulty hearing faint speech in noise
Mild	Difficulty hearing faint or distant speech, even in quiet
Moderate	Hears conversational speech only at a close distance
Moderately severe	Hears loud conversational speech
Severe	Cannot hear conversational speech
Profound	May hear loud sounds; hearing is not the primary communication channel

Source: Data from Stach, B. A. (1998). Clinical audiology: An introduction. Clifton Park, NY: Thomson Delmar Learning. Adapted by permission.

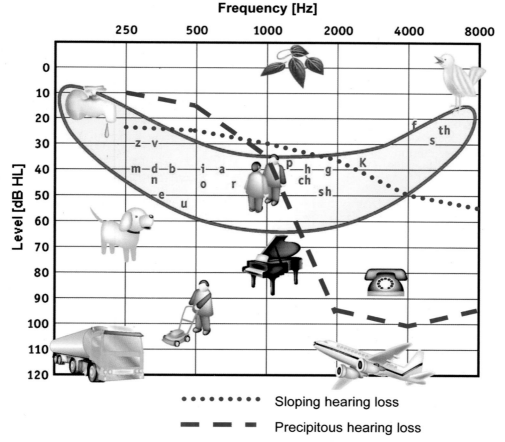

Figure 2–5   Sound sources and hearing losses. Illustration created by Lerch Design Studio. Copyright by Bernafon AG. Reprinted by permission.

with levels below their hearing loss curves). For instance, the sloping hearing loss makes the sibilants inaudible, while the precipitous hearing loss also affects stop consonants.

Consonants generally have a lower short-term sound pressure level than vowels. Nevertheless, they are important for understanding speech. The effect is familiar: hearing-impaired persons often misunderstand what is said because they confuse the softer consonants.

Impact on Hearing Aid Design

Hearing loss differs in *shape* and *degree*, as we have seen in the Hearing Loss section. And the *loudness growth function* described in the same-named section revealed the *recruitment* effect: *sensorineural* hearing loss makes it necessary to amplify soft sounds more than loud sounds to restore normal loudness perception. In some cases, hearing-impaired persons perceive sounds at high sound pressure levels even louder than listeners with normal hearing. All of these findings translate into requirements to a hearing aid. It must provide flexible programming, and it must

◆ Allow different amplification at different frequencies

◆ Be able to amplify soft sounds more than loud ones

◆ Avoid producing painfully loud sound by limiting the maximum output level

◆ Summary

In this chapter, we first looked at the hearing loss – at its different types, degrees, and configurations. The next two sections dealt with the loudness growth function and with speech audiometry. Finally, we looked at how hearing impairment affects hearing and understanding speech, and how it impacts hearing aid design.

References

American National Standards Institute. (1996). ANSI S3.6, American National Standard Specification for audiometers. Washington, DC: American National Standards Institute.

Brand, T., and Hohmann, V. (2002). An adaptive procedure for categorical loudness scaling, Journal of the Acoustical Society of America, 112(4), 1597–1604.

Dillon, H. (2001). Hearing aids. New York: Thieme Medical Publishers.

Elberling, C. (1999). Loudness scaling revisited. Journal of the American Academy of Audiology, 10(5), 248–260.

Gelfand, S. A. (2001). Essentials of audiology. New York: Thieme Medical Publishers.

International Electrotechnical Commission. (1985). IEC 60268-1, Sound system equipment, Part 1: General (2nd ed.). Geneva: International Electrotechnical Commission.

Kalikow, D. N., Stevens, K. N., and Elliott, L. L. (1977). Development of a test of speech intelligibility in noise using sentence materials with controlled word predictability. Journal of the Acoustical Society of America, 61(5), 1337–1351.

Katz, J. (2001). Handbook of clinical audiology (5th ed.). Baltimore, MD: Lippincott Williams & Wilkins.

Kiessling, J., Schubert, M., and Archut, A. (1996). Adaptive fitting of hearing instruments by category loudness scaling (ScalAdapt). Scandinavian Audiology, 25(3), 153–160.

Nilsson, M., Soli, S. D., and Sullivan, J. (1994). Development of a hearing in noise test for the measurement of speech reception threshold, Journal of the Acoustical Society of America, 95(2), 1085–1099.

Roeser, R. J., Valente, M., and Hosford-Dunn, H. (2000). Audiology: Diagnosis. New York: Thieme Medical Publishers.

Roeser, R. J., Valente, M., and Hosford-Dunn, H. (2000). Audiology: Treatment. New York: Thieme Medical Publishers.

Sataloff, R. T., and Sataloff, J. (1993). Hearing loss. New York: Marcel Dekker.

Stach, B. A. (1998). Clinical audiology: An introduction. Clifton Park, NY: Thomson Delmar Learning.

3

Overview of Hearing Aid Characteristics

This chapter addresses three topics:

1. *Customer satisfaction*: What factors will most likely satisfy the customer's needs?
2. *Hearing aid styles*: What are the main options regarding the physical style of today's hearing instruments?
3. *The impact of digital technology*: How much does digital signal processing contribute to customer satisfaction?

Topics 1 and 3 are controversial – and this book will not resolve these issues. It will instead demonstrate how digital signal processing works in today's hearing instruments, and cite references to sources that express different opinions.

◆ Customer Satisfaction

A survey (Kochkin, 2005) of more than 1,500 users of hearing instruments measured 71% overall satisfaction with instruments that are 0 to 5 years old, and 78% with 1-year-old instruments. This result puts hearing instruments in the top third of all products and services listed in the *American Customer Satisfaction Index*, as measured by the University of Michigan.

The survey analyzed which factors influence customer satisfaction the most. **Table 3–1** summarizes the findings; the higher the number ρ, the more the factor affects customer satisfaction. In essence, the important factors boil down to four areas: sound quality, speech intelligibility, reliability, and cost.

The analysis also revealed what factors impact customer satisfaction the least. **Table 3–2** shows

the result; the lower the number ρ, the less the factor affects customer satisfaction. The findings in **Table 3–2** hold a surprise: *visibility of the hearing instrument* ranks lowest on correlation with overall satisfaction. Nevertheless, this feature has considerably driven the development of hearing aids, as we will see from the next section about hearing aid styles.

Other opinions contrast with Kochkin's survey. Killion (2004), for instance, completely denies a link between customer satisfaction and benefit. He instead claims that the public believes in six commonly accepted myths:

Myth #1 Significant technology improvements will consistently increase expressed satisfaction with hearing aids.

Myth #2 Increased benefit always results in increased patient satisfaction.

Myth #3 Increased hearing aid cost increases perceived value.

Myth #4 First-fit algorithms provide sufficient gain to make quiet speech understandable.

Myth #5 The gain and frequency response on the computer screen is what the hearing aid is delivering to your patient.

Myth #6 Hearing aid fitting and adjustment by a professional will always increase patient satisfaction above the level of an aid that is not professionally fitted.

To each myth, the author elaborates extensive arguments. Given that the technical advancements are limited, myths #4 and #5 make it clear how important it is to carry out verification tests.

Table 3–1   Factors that Relate Most with Customer Satisfaction

Rank	Factor	ρ*
1	Overall benefit	0.74
2	Clarity of sound	0.72
3	Value†	0.69
4	Reliability of the hearing instrument	0.69
5	Natural sounding	0.68
6	Ability to hear in small groups	0.66
7	Richness of fidelity of sound	0.64
8	One-to-one conversation	0.63
9	Leisure activities	0.63
10	Listening to TV	0.62

Source: Data from Kochkin, S. (2005). Customer satisfaction with hearing instruments in the digital age. The Hearing Journal, 58(9): 30–43.
*ρ denotes the correlation with overall hearing instrument satisfaction.
†Value denotes the performance of the hearing instrument relative to price.

Table 3–2   Factors that Relate Least with Customer Satisfaction

Rank	Factor	ρ*
1	Visibility of hearing instrument	0.34
2	Hearing instrument usage: hours worn	0.36
3	Front office staff	0.38
4	Ease of changing battery	0.41
5	Battery life	0.41
6	Ease of adjusting volume	0.44
7	Dispenser service	0.46
8	Packaging	0.48

Source: Data from Kochkin, S. (2005). Customer satisfaction with hearing instruments in the digital age. The Hearing Journal, 58(9): 30–43.
*ρ denotes the correlation with overall hearing instrument satisfaction.

◆ Hearing Aid Styles

The term style refers to the physical size of a hearing instrument, to what it looks like, and to where it is worn. **Figure 3–1** shows the six currently most popular options, from left to right:

1. A completely-in-the-canal hearing aid (CIC)
2. An in-the-canal hearing aid (ITC)
3. An in-the-ear hearing aid (ITE)

4. A behind-the-ear hearing aid (BTE) with standard tubing and custom earmold
5. A behind-the-ear hearing aid (BTE) with thin tube and dome
6. A behind-the-ear hearing aid with the receiver in the ear (RITE) canal

The BTE with standard tubing and custom earmold is the oldest of the styles shown. ITE, ITC, and CIC instruments gradually emerged, as hearing aid components became smaller and smaller. Their major advantage is purely cosmetic, especially the CIC instruments. The BTE with thin tube and dome as well as with the

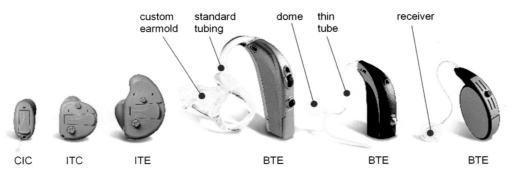

Figure 3–1   Different hearing aid styles.

receiver in the ear canal have recently completed the range. Their main advantage is wearing comfort because they leave the ear canal open—hence the technical term *open fitting*.

The custom-made earmold is part of the sound conducting mechanism of the traditional BTE fitting. It seals up the ear canal and provides a bore for the sound from the receiver to travel via the tube and through the earmold into the ear canal. There is no need for an earmold with CIC, ITC, and ITE instruments. They are also custom-made and fit closely in the ear canal as well.

Completely blocking up the ear canal, however, causes the *occlusion effect*: the wearer's own voice sounds louder and hollow, while breathing and chewing sounds sound considerably louder. This is because, in addition to the sound waves carried through the air, the bones of the skull also transmit sound. When the ear canal is open, the additional sound flows out unnoticed, but cannot do so if the ear is blocked. To prevent the occlusion effect, the earmold usually provides an additional bore in parallel to the sound channel: the *vent*. Besides its effect on the acoustics, the vent also avoids excessive moisture buildup in the ear canal and relieves pressure while inserting and removing the hearing instrument.

Hearing instruments fitted into the ear canal usually have a built-in vent, and BTE instruments with thin tube and dome or with the receiver in the ear canal already leave the ear canal open. The more open the ear canal remains, however, the more amplified sound gets out of the ear canal and the more direct sound from the free field gets in. Hence large vents and open fittings have two consequences; they

- Increase the tendency for acoustic feedback
- Reduce the benefit of advanced features such as noise reduction and possibly acoustic directionality as well

The hearing aid style also impacts the use of local controls. BTE and ITE instruments offer enough space to provide for a rotary wheel and for a push button; so, the hearing aid user can adjust sound intensity and change hearing programs in different sound environments. A CIC instrument, however, usually requires a remote control to accomplish this.

As a result, there is no ideal style; each style has its advantages and disadvantages – see Dillon (2001) for further discussion of hearing instrument styles.

◆ The Impact of Digital Technology

The introduction to the survey (Kochkin, 2005) states that digital hearing instruments offer eight significant advantages that were not available before with analog hearing instruments:

1. Superior signal processing (DSP) capabilities, increasing the chances that noise sources will be removed and that the instrument will capture and understand more of the speech signal, or that some sounds will be enhanced to aid speech intelligibility.

2. Active noise reduction and cancellation and therefore greater user comfort in noisy situations.

3. Greater flexibility in fitting the instrument to the unique hearing loss characteristics of the consumer.

4. Better ability to reduce internal noise in the hearing instrument through suppression of acoustic and mechanical feedback.

5. Superior optimization of microphones in directional hearing instruments.

6. Better overall shaping of the frequency response.

7. The ability, through data logging, to use DSP to better monitor hearing instrument use, which will aid the fine-tuning process for some consumers.

8. Overall cleaner sound delivered to the consumer's ears.

These statements are based on numerous references (Westermann & Sandlin, 1997; Powers & Wesselkamp, 1999; Agnew, 1999; Mueller, 2000; Mueller, 2002; Smith & Levitt, 2000) and reinforced by a double-blinded study (Schum & Pogash, 2003) that compared three levels of hearing instrument technology. In this comparison, 74% of the consumers rated a second-generation digital hearing instrument significantly higher than both an analog and a first-generation digital hearing instrument.

As mentioned at the beginning of this chapter, the digital advantage is controversial. Other studies either found the digital advantage to be less impressive (Wood & Lutman, 2004), or that the advantage only matters little in everyday life (Walden et al, 2000; Newman & Sandridge,

1998). Later chapters will contain more references addressing specific topics that relate to the technology used in digital hearing instruments.

The remaining parts of this section will present an introduction to the various signal processing algorithms that bring about the digital advantage in current hearing instruments:

◆ *Digital amplification* provides better overall shaping of the frequency response, including greater flexibility in fitting the hearing instrument to the unique hearing loss characteristics of the hearing-impaired person

◆ *Acoustic directionality* provides superior optimization of microphones in directional hearing instruments, increasing the chances that noise sources will be removed

◆ *Noise reduction* provides greater user comfort in noisy situations

◆ *Feedback cancellation* reduces acoustic and mechanical feedback

◆ *Sound classification* provides greater user comfort by analyzing the acoustic signal and adapting the signal processing to the different listening environments

Each of these topics deserves more than just an introduction. Chapters 4 to 10 will present them in detail.

Digital Amplification

In the previous chapter, we looked at the issues of sensorineural hearing loss and recruitment. Intuition suggests amplifying soft sounds by more and loud sounds by less – to compensate for the abnormal loudness growth. The technical term for this amplification strategy is *wide dynamic range compression* (WDRC). Although its logic seems compelling, WDRC does not work for everybody. In the study by Schum and Pogash (2003), all test persons had sensorineural hearing loss. As mentioned before, the study reports significant advantages for the digital technology, but still 10% of the test persons preferred linear amplification (i.e., the same gain for sounds of all input levels).

Nevertheless, WDRC requires more flexibility from a hearing instrument than linear amplification does. We will therefore look at how analog and digital technology succeed in realizing WDRC. **Figure 3–2** shows an example of target gain curves that the present-day National Acoustic Laboratories–Non-Linear 1 (NAL-NL1) fitting rationale (Dillon, 1999; Keidser et al, 1999) derived for a sloping hearing loss.

The diagram shows *in-situ gain* for input signals of 50, 60, 70, 80 and 90 dB SPL. The *in-situ gain* is the difference between the sound level at the tympanic membrane and that at free

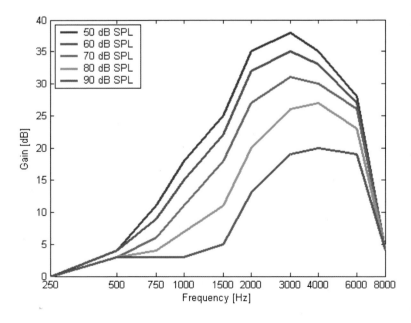

Figure 3–2 Target gain for wide dynamic range compression.

field. In this example, NAL-NL1 recommends 20 dB less gain at 3 kHz when the input level is 90 dB SPL instead of 50 dB SPL.

In Chapter 4, we will look at amplification schemes that were already implemented in analog hearing instruments. The focus will be on the flexibility the different schemes provide to fit to the given amplification targets. In Chapter 5, we will see how various digital amplification schemes perform on the same task.

WDRC also has temporal behavior: how fast does a hearing instrument reduce gain, when the input level increases? And how fast does it again increase amplification, when the input level decreases? Chapter 6 will discuss the temporal behavior.

Acoustic Directionality

Hearing-impaired persons often complain that they cannot understand speech well in an acoustically difficult surrounding—in background conversational babble or in background noise at work. Just as they miss certain sounds or phonemes because of their hearing loss, background noise can also mask the signal components in parts of the frequency spectrum.

A directional microphone can help if the background noise and the desired signal come from different directions – noise from the side or from behind, for example. **Figure 3–3** illustrates

the situation by showing the polar directivity pattern of various microphone types. Using polar coordinates, this diagram displays along the radius how sensitive the various microphones are for sound approaching from all angles, from 0 degrees front direction to 180 degrees back direction. The microphones are matched so that they feature equal sensitivity in the 0-degree viewing direction. At angles of +90 degrees and −90 degrees, only the *omnidirectional* directivity pattern still has the same sensitivity, whereas the various *cardioid* patterns already attenuate by 6, 9, and 12 dB to the side.

Cardioids, supercardioids, and *hypercardioids* are all insensitive to sounds coming from a certain angle (Thompson, 2005; Gibbon et al, 1997). **Table 3–3** shows these *null directions.* Normal microphones have *omnidirectional* characteristics—they are equally sensitive to sounds from all directions and thus have no *null direction.*

Table 3–3 shows a further property of directional microphones: the *directivity index* (Blauert, 2005; Valente 2002). This index describes the spatial sensitivity, illustrated in **Fig. 3–4**. The different forms are obtained by rotating the curves in **Fig. 3–3**, taking the wearer's viewing direction as the axis of rotation.

The directivity index quantifies how much a directional microphone improves the *signal-to-noise ratio* for a signal coming from the front,

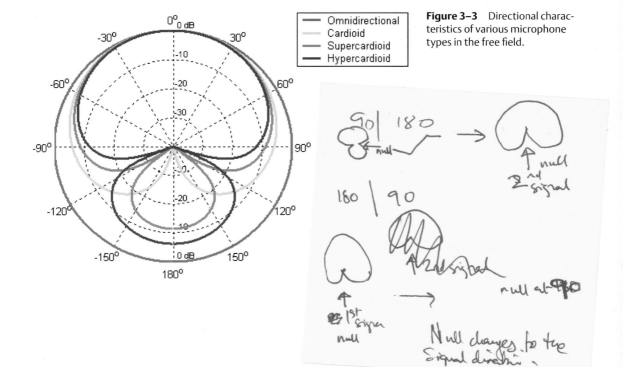

Omnidirectional
Cardioid
Supercardioid
Hypercardioid

Figure 3–3   Directional characteristics of various microphone types in the free field.

Table 3–3 Null Direction and Directivity Index for Various Directional Patterns

Directional Characteristic	Null Direction	Directivity Index (DI)
Omnidirectional	None	0.0 dB
Cardioid	180°	4.8 dB
Supercardioid	±125°	5.7 dB
Hypercardioid	±110°	6.0 dB

Source: Data from (1) Blauert, J. (2005). Communication acoustics. New York/Heidelberg/Berlin: Springer. (2) Gibbon, D., Moore, R., and Winski, R. (1997). Handbook of standards and resources for spoken language systems. New York: Walter de Gruyter. (3) Thompson, D. M. (2005). Understanding audio: Getting the most out of your project or professional recording studio. Indianapolis, IN: Hal Leonard. (4) Valente, M. (2002). Hearing aids: Standards, options, and limitations (2nd ed.). New York: Thieme Medical Publishers.

compared with sounds from all other directions.

Example: A desired signal arrives from the 0-degree direction with a certain sound pressure level, while background noise arrives from all other directions with the same total level.

If an omnidirectional microphone receives these signals, then the signal to noise ratio will be 0 dB. A directional microphone with a *hypercardioid* characteristic, however, will attenuate

the background noise level by around 6 dB, resulting in a signal to noise ratio of 6 dB.

The characteristics shown in **Fig. 3–3, Fig. 3–4**, and **Table 3–3** are only strictly valid for the ideal case, where the microphone is placed in free field, or in an anechoic room. Wearing a hearing aid with a directional microphone in a normal living room or office makes a difference. Room reflections and the way sound travels around the head will lead to different behavior, and in particular, to a lower directivity index.

As Walden et al (2000) report in their study, directional microphones indeed produce different results under ideal test conditions and in everyday life. In an anechoic test room, the sound energy from a sound source reaches a hearing instrument via the direct path. In a reverberant room, however, a listener receives direct sound energy as well as reflected sound energy. The farther away a listener is from a target speaker in this case, the less direct sound energy and the more reflected sound energy will reach him or her. The same also holds for a distant noise source in the rear hemisphere: the farther away the source is, the less sound energy approaches from a specific angle and the more sound energy arrives from all around. As a result, directional microphones will provide less and less benefit.

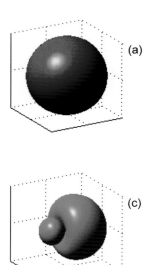

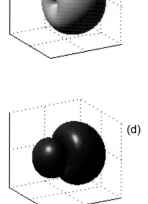

Figure 3–4 Spatial representation of directional characteristics: **(a)** omnidirectional, **(b)** cardioid, **(c)** supercardioid, and **(d)** hypercardioid.

A technical concept captures the situation: the *critical distance*; it is the distance from a sound source at which the two sound energies equal each other. Within critical distance, a listener gets at least half of the sound energy via the direct path and directional microphones provide a useful benefit. The value of the critical distance depends on the size of a room and on how much the room reverberates; in a living room the critical distance is typically 1 to 2 m and may extend to 5 m in large halls.

Directional microphones have already been used in analog hearing aids. Processing the signal digitally, however, adds two advantages: *adaptive* directionality and processing in subbands. The *adaptive* processing constantly moves the null direction to track and cancel the strongest signal from the rear hemisphere. This proves helpful, when the noise from the rear hemisphere is direct sound energy, rather than arriving evenly from all directions. Processing the acoustic signal in separate frequency bands helps canceling multiple noise sources, given their signals differ significantly in spectral contents.

Chapter 7 will go into more detail and show how acoustic directionality works in today's hearing instruments.

Noise Reduction

Hearing-impaired persons appreciate a hearing aid that applies an intelligent strategy to process speech, music, and noise in different ways. In Chapter 1 (Everyday Acoustic Signals). we have seen how much the properties of various everyday signals differ from one another. Recognizing these differences enables a hearing instrument to adaptively suppress noise. For this purpose the instrument analyzes the signal in separate frequency bands, and attenuates the band signals that contain mainly noise. In this way the instrument attempts to minimize auditory fatigue.

To better understand the background of this strategy we will take a quick look at the *speech intelligibility index* (American National Standards Institute, 1997), abbreviated to SII. With a value between 0 and 1 the index indicates the proportion of speech cues that are available to a listener in a specific situation.

To reach the maximum index value of 1 requires two conditions to be fulfilled in each of the analysis frequency bands:

1. The level of the speech signal must not be more than 10 dB above the level of normal speech when spoken from a distance of 1 m.

   Amplifying loud signals less may therefore slightly improve the index, and speech should consequently become slightly more understandable – according to the SII model.

2. The level of the speech signal must exceed the noise level by at least 15 dB.

This second condition gives rise to the *15-dB rule*:

Let X be the signal to noise ratio in some frequency band and assume $X < 15$ dB. Then, it is possible to amplify that band signal less by $(15 - X)$ dB without reducing the index score.

Example: signal to noise ratio = 11 dB → amplify by 4 dB less, as $15 - 11 = 4$.

What is the reason behind this *15-dB rule*? Amplification tends to raise signals at least 15 dB over the hearing threshold to assure intelligibility, again according to the SII model. The hearing instrument, however, amplifies both the signal and the noise in equal measure. So, even if the signal gets just 15 dB above threshold, the noise is also 4 dB above threshold in our example. And reducing the gain by 4 dB thus pushes the noise back closer to threshold, while still keeping the useful signal above.

Normally, both the desired signal and the unwanted noise are present at the same time, thus preventing an instrument from measuring their levels separately. In this instance, a hearing aid uses *modulation* instead. Modulation designates the difference between the largest and smallest levels observed over a short time interval.

Adaptively reducing noise can be compared with a tone control that either allows the signal to pass through in certain frequency bands, or attenuates it by a larger or smaller amount, depending on the modulation. **Figure 3–5** shows two examples:

◆ **Figure 3–5a** shows the effect of a noise reduction algorithm in the presence of low-frequency noise. In this case, the noise reduction acts as a high-pass filter and prevents the low-frequency noise from masking parts of the wanted signal at high frequencies.

◆ **Figure 3–5b**, on the other hand, shows how the adaptive processing affects a signal that contains high frequency noise. In this case,

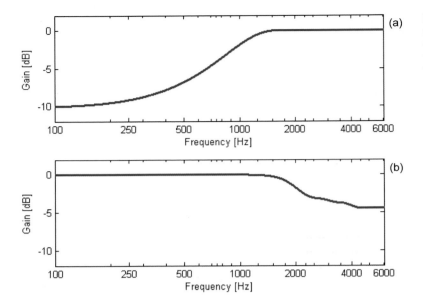

Figure 3–5   Effect of noise reduction in the presence of different signals: **(a)** low-frequency noise, and **(b)** high-frequency noise.

the noise reduction acts as a low-pass filter and suppresses the high-frequency noise.

Chapter 8 will go into more details and will show how noise reduction works in today's hearing instruments.

Feedback Cancellation

Various factors increase the risk that a hearing aid will begin to whistle: high gain, small physical size, a poorly fit earmold or instrument case, a large vent, open fitting, cerumen in the ear canal, etc. A hearing aid begins to whistle when amplified sound feeds back from the receiver to the microphone with a greater level than when it reached the microphone the first time. The signal then passes through the instrument again and again, each time undergoing additional amplification, until finally it reaches the maximum output level.

Normally, when an instrument whistles, a single sinusoidal signal component dominates; but sometimes more than one is present simultaneously. This depends on how sound spreads out in the vicinity of the hearing instrument and where reflections occur.

When an analog hearing instrument whistles, there is no alternative to reducing amplification at the critical frequencies. Most digital hearing aids suppress feedback differently;

they amplify as usual and suppress the feedback adaptively with the type of processing shown in **Fig. 3–6**.

The blue arrow indicates the route that sound takes from the free field to the tympanic membrane. The red arrow indicates the feedback signal that causes the hearing aid to whistle when the path from the receiver to the microphone attenuates insufficiently.

The feedback model in **Fig. 3–6** continuously estimates the signal that feeds back from the receiver to the microphone. The model also adjusts itself whenever something changes in the vicinity of the hearing aid, thereby influencing the sound on its way back to the microphone. In the ideal case, subtracting the estimated value from the microphone signal causes only the sound from the free field to remain. The hearing aid subsequently processes this clean signal and transmits it via the receiver to the tympanic membrane. In practice, adaptive feedback cancellation achieves an additional gain margin of around 10 dB. What does this mean?

Example: Assume a hearing aid is programmed in such a way that it does not normally whistle, but starts to whistle as soon as the wearer brings a telephone receiver to his or her ear. Turning an adaptive feedback canceller on will then prevent the hearing aid from

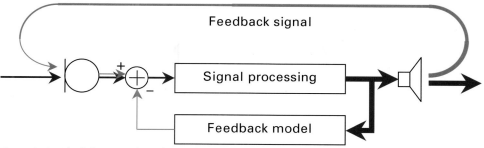

Figure 3–6   Block diagram of an adaptive feedback canceller.

whistling in the same situation, even though the gain is the same as before.

Chapter 9 will go into more details and will show how feedback cancellation works in today's hearing instruments.

Sound Classification

The variety of everyday acoustic signals is enormous. In Chapter 1, we have seen that they can be broadly divided into three categories: speech, music, and noise.

As **Fig. 3–7** indicates, hearing-impaired persons will benefit from a hearing aid that changes its mode of operation to process signals from different signal categories in different ways.

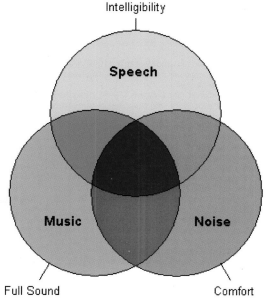

Figure 3–7   Different amplification targets for different signal categories.

♦ For *speech* the hearing aid should, above all, promote the mid and high frequencies, and cautiously amplify low-frequency sounds. This guideline is a component of today's fitting algorithms such as NAL-NL1. The targets are set this way for maximum speech intelligibility.

♦ Strong low-frequency signal components give *music* presence; a broadband amplification generates a full and impressive sound.

♦ For *noise* signals the situation is different again. Monotonic noise in particular creates auditory fatigue. However, pulsed sounds such as the clattering of plates and cutlery are also tiring for hearing-impaired listeners. In both cases they want their hearing aids to amplify these sounds less than music and speech.

In the Noise Reduction subsection above, we considered noise reduction and found a rule: the lower the amount of modulation present in a frequency band, the more attenuation the noise reduction system applies to that band signal. This works effectively in the case of monotonic noise, such as the train noise discussed in Chapter 1 for example. There the signal level is more or less constant in all frequency bands, the modulation is thus small, and so the noise-reduction system attenuates the entire noise. However, taking a closer look reveals that noise reduction typically fails in two cases, pulsed noise and music.

1. *Pulsed noise:* in the clattering crockery signal also discussed in Chapter 1, the amplitude of the sound pressure oscillations – and with it the sound pressure level – repeatedly increases in large steps, and decreases again as soon as the sound dies away. This behavior causes the

signal to have significant modulation in all frequency bands, preventing the noise reduction system from attenuating the noise.

2. *Music* often contains tone sequences at more or less a constant level, in other words with low modulation. This can affect the whole frequency range, as in the example of easy listening music discussed in Chapter 1, or single bands as in the low-frequency area of the classical music extract discussed in the same section in Chapter 1. This occasionally low modulation leads the noise reduction system to repeatedly attenuate the whole signal or in just some bands, and then to remove the attenuation again. This behavior is annoying when listening closely to music.

The examples give an idea of how difficult it is to automatically control a hearing aid correctly all the time. If sound classification works correctly, it will be capable of fixing the shortcomings of traditional noise reduction schemes. But it offers even more potential: it enables hearing aids to adapt all of its features to the particular listening situation, including the gain as mentioned before, but also acoustic directionality and feedback cancellation.

By relieving their users of manual program changes and volume adjustments, a hearing aid allows wearers to concentrate on the acoustic signal and is thus likely to improve their quality of life. The key to automatic program selection lies with sampling and evaluating enough signal attributes to sufficiently characterize the acoustic signals. Such features include sound pressure level and modulation, and extend to periodicity, spectral envelopes, and more.

Two factors further complicate the task:

1. As **Fig. 3–7** illustrates, there are often multiple sound sources present simultaneously. This makes it more difficult to reliably identify the listening situation and to make the correct processing decision, for example with speech in noise.

2. Even if a hearing aid analyzes a lot of signal attributes, its decisions are still built on a statistical basis. Hence it will still occasionally allocate a signal to the wrong category.

In everyday life, sound classification is correct in ~80% typically. Hearing aids therefore still allow the wearer to manually select a program and adjust sound intensity, and thereby override an automatic setting.

Chapter 10 will go more into detail and sketch the basics of sound classification.

◆ Summary

This chapter first addressed the factors that most likely impact satisfaction with hearing instruments. It then presented a brief overview of hearing aid styles and went on to discuss the advantages of digital technology. The focus finally was on introducing the various digital signal processing algorithms that today's hearing instruments offer: digital amplification, acoustic directionality, noise reduction, feedback cancellation, and sound classification.

References

Agnew, J. (1999). Challenges and some solutions for understanding speech in noise, high performance hearing solutions. Hearing Review, 3, 4–9.

American National Standards Institute. (1997) ANSI S3.5 - R2002: American National Standard methods for calculation of the speech intelligibility index. Washington, DC: American National Standards Institute.

Blauert, J. (2005). Communication acoustics. New York/Heidelberg/Berlin: Springer.

Dillon, H. (1999). NAL-NL1: A new prescriptive fitting procedure for non-linear hearing aids. The Hearing Journal, 52(4), 10–16.

Dillon, H. (2001). Hearing aids. New York: Thieme Medical Publishers.

Gibbon, D., Moore, R., and Winski, R. (1997). Handbook of standards and resources for spoken language systems. New York: Walter de Gruyter.

Keidser G., Dillon H., and Brewer S. (1999). Using the NAL-NL1 prescriptive procedure with advanced hearing instruments. The Hearing Review, 6(11), 8–20.

Killion, M. C. (2004, August): Myths about hearing aid benefit and satisfaction. The Hearing Review, pp. 14, 16, 18–20, 66.

Kochkin, S. (2005). Customer satisfaction with hearing instruments in the digital age. The Hearing Journal, 58(9), 30–43.

Mueller H. G. (2000). What's the digital difference when it comes to patient benefit? The Hearing Journal, 53(3), 23–32.

Mueller H. G. (2002). A candid round-table discussion on modern digital hearing aids and their features. The Hearing Journal, 55(10), 23–35.

Newman, C.W., and Sandridge, S. A. (1998): Benefit from, satisfaction with, and cost-effectiveness of three different hearing aid technologies. American Journal of Audiology, 7, 115–128.

Powers, T., and Wesselkamp, M. (1999). The use of digital features to combat background noise. Hearing Review, 3, 36–39.

Schum, D. J., and Pogash, R. R. (2003). Blinded comparison of three levels of hearing aid technology. The Hearing Review, 10(1), 40–43, 64–65.

Smith, L. Z., and Levitt, H. (2000). Improving speech recognition in children: New hopes with digital hearing aids. The Hearing Journal, 53(3), 70–74.

Thompson, D. M. (2005). Understanding audio: Getting the most out of your project or professional recording studio. Indianapolis, IN: Hal Leonard.

Valente, M. (2002). Hearing aids: Standards, options, and limitations (2nd ed.). New York: Thieme Medical Publishers.

Walden, B. E., Surr, R. K., Cord, M. T., Edwards B., and Olson, L. (2000). Comparison of benefits provided by different hearing aid technologies. Journal of the American Academy of Audiology, 11(10), 540–560.

Westermann, S., and Sandlin, R. E. (1997). Digital signal processing: Benefits and expectations, high performance hearing solutions (Vol. 2). Hearing Review, 4(suppl 11), 56–59.

Wood, S. A., and Lutman, M. E. (2004). Relative benefits of linear analogue and advanced digital hearing aids. International Journal of Audiology, 43(3), 144–155.

4

Basic Amplification Schemes

This chapter consists of five sections. The first and second sections address basic questions about amplification in hearing aids; the next three sections present amplification schemes that were implemented previously in analog hearing instruments. Briefly the questions addressed and the topics presented are

1. What are the *objectives of wide dynamic range compression* (WDRC)?
2. Besides electronic amplification, what other *effects on the acoustic signal* are present as sound travels from the free field to the tympanic membrane?
3. *Linear hearing instrument*: provides constant gain for sounds of all input levels.
4. *Broadband compression*: the shape of the gain curve is fixed; gain varies uniformly across frequency.
5. *Two-channel WDRC*: varies gain separately in two frequency channels.

Studies that compare WDRC versus linear amplification usually find that both methods provide significant benefit. The differences between methods are smaller and lead to equivocal results. Larson et al (2000), for instance, report patients' order of preference as follows: linear amplification with compression limiting (41.6%), WDRC (29.8%), and linear amplification with peak-clipping (28.6%). Humes et al (1999), on the other hand, report that WDRC instruments are superior to linear devices for many outcome measures.

As mentioned in the previous chapter, the focus here is on exploring the flexibility that the processing schemes offer to fit the unique hearing loss of each individual. The methods described in this chapter were already applied in analog technology. The next chapter will present what digital technology has brought about. For a more detailed discussion, see Venema (2006) and Dillon (2001).

◆ Objectives of Wide Dynamic Range Compression

WDRC aims to compensate for the abnormal loudness growth that affects hearing-impaired people with sensorineural hearing loss. To accomplish this, WDRC amplifies soft sounds by more and loud sounds by less. Although the approach seems clear, strategies differ in

◆ Defining the amount of gain to apply
◆ How fast to react when the sound pressure level of the input signal changes

Today's hearing aids should, however, be flexible enough to meet the amplification targets regardless of the guiding principle behind a fitting strategy. They should also prove to be flexible enough to provide for all potential changes in subsequent fine-tuning sessions. Exploring this fitting flexibility forms the topic of this and the next chapter.

Differences in Defining Gain

Prescribing gain usually follows one of two principles:

1. Loudness normalization aims at amplifying sounds at every level and frequency so that

a hearing-impaired person perceives the amplified sound to be at the same loudness as a listener with normal hearing.

2. Maximizing speech intelligibility is the objective of the present-day National Acoustic Laboratories—Non-Linear 1 (NAL-NL1) fitting algorithm (Dillon, 1999; Keidser et al, 1999) – with a consequence on loudness: a hearing-impaired person shall perceive amplified speech to be, at most, the same loudness that a listener with normal hearing would perceive the original speech signal.

In achieving its aim, NAL-NL1 tends to prescribe gain that amplifies normal speech to equal loudness levels across frequency (Keidser & Grant, 2003) – hence the term *loudness equalization* to distinguish NAL-NL1 from fitting procedures that are based on *loudness normalization*, such as the IHAFF (independent hearing aid fitting forum) fitting rationale (Valente & Van Vliet, 1997), for example.

Differences in Reacting to Changes in Sound Pressure Level

Implementations of WDRC usually reduce gain quickly, when the sound pressure level of the input signal rises. In this way they prevent signal overshoot (i.e., they avoid emitting too loud output signals). When the sound level goes down, however, implementations show a wide span of reaction times to again increase amplification:

◆ The *automatic volume control* only gradually increases gain. As a result, the hearing instrument only follows the *peak value* when the sound pressure level of a signal changes continuously between large and small values, as with speech for example. The instrument only adjusts itself slowly when it passes from a loud environment into a quiet one; this may take up to several seconds.

◆ *Syllabic compression* increases gain more quickly, when the sound pressure level of the input signal goes down. As the name implies, syllabic compression aims at dealing separately with each syllable in running speech.

Studies on the speed of WDRC report equivocal results: Hansen (2002) finds best speech intelligibility and sound quality with slow-acting multi-channel WDRC; release time = 4

seconds. Bentler and Duve (2000) report no difference in speech perception measures for a variety of WDRC systems that featured temporal behavior from automatic volume control to syllabic compression. Marriage and Moore (2003) report that moderate-to-profound children significantly benefit from fast-acting WDRC as compared with linear amplification. The different population may, of course, have an influence.

Chapter 6 will present the temporal behavior of WDRC, covering compression speed from slow to very fast.

◆ Effects on the Acoustic Signal

Thinking about hearing aid amplification usually focuses on the electronic module. This is the part that amplifies the acoustic signal differently for each hearing-impaired person, thus compensating for the individual's hearing loss. Apart from the electronic module, many other elements amplify or attenuate the sound on its way from the free field to the tympanic membrane. We will look first at the effect of the outer ear, when no hearing aid is present. Then we will consider what happens when a hearing-impaired person wears an instrument in his or her ear canal.

By the Outer Ear

The outer ear – the combination of the pinna and the external ear canal – amplifies sound waves as they travel from the free field to the tympanic membrane, and it does so by different amounts at different frequencies. **Figure 4–1** shows this *open ear response* for an adult, in the frequency range between 250 Hz and 8 kHz.

The technical term for such a gain curve is *transfer function*.

Definition: For a system that transmits signals – in our example the outer ear – the *transfer function* defines how much the system amplifies or attenuates at each frequency.

Due to differences in ear size and shape, the *open ear response* is different for every individual; however, it generally rises with increasing frequency up to ~3 kHz, where it reaches a peak of ~15 dB, and then falls.

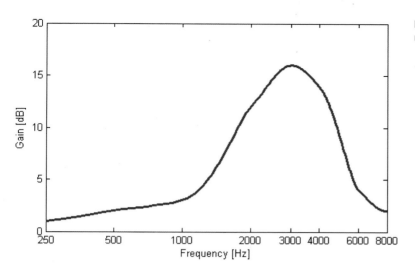

Figure 4–1   The open ear response of an adult.

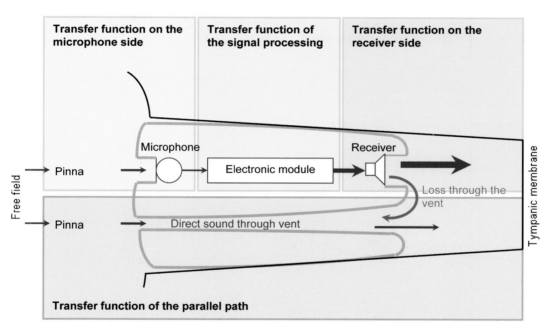

Figure 4–2   A schematic cross-section of a hearing instrument in the ear canal.

By an Instrument in the Ear Canal

Figure 4–2 shows a diagrammatic cross-section of an ear canal that contains a hearing instrument with a built-in vent. There are two signal paths from the free field to the tympanic membrane in this case. Along the main path the hearing aid amplifies the free field sound, while the sound also passes directly into the

ear canal via the vent. And at the same time, amplified sound also leaves the ear canal via the vent.

Table 4–1 summarizes the various effects and makes it clear: the programmable electronic module is only one of several factors. The focus here is on exploring all factors except the electronic module. So, let us assume that the electronic module acts as an all-pass filter,

Table 4–1   Effects on the Acoustic Signal

Signal Path	Element	Transfer Function
Main path	Pinna Microphone	Transfer function on the microphone side
	Electronic module	Signal processing transfer function
	Receiver Vent	Transfer function on the receiver side
Parallel path	Pinna Vent	Transfer function of the parallel path

just like a wire between the microphone and the receiver. With this assumption in mind, we will consider the transfer functions:

- On the microphone side
- On the receiver side – including the vent with regards to sound leaving the ear canal
- Of the parallel path, including the vent with regards to sound entering the ear canal
- Of the combination of these three factors – from now on referred to as *basic gain*

Then we conclude with an additional effect:

- Insertion loss

Transfer Function on the Microphone Side

Figure 4–3a shows a transfer function on the microphone side. It is made up of two parts:

1. The transfer function of the pinna. This amplifies less than the whole outer ear (pinna and external ear canal combined), but still cannot be neglected.
2. The microphone transfer function

The microphone transfer function depends strongly on the particular microphone type. The model in our example amplifies more as the frequency increases, until it reaches a maximum of ~5 dB at around 5 kHz. Together with the pinna this results in a transfer function achieving slightly more than 10 dB at 5 kHz.

Transfer Function on the Receiver Side

Figure 4–3b shows a transfer function on the receiver side. It is also made up of two parts:

1. The receiver transfer function
2. The effect of the vent on sound that leaves the ear canal

The receiver transfer function again depends on the particular type. In this example, the

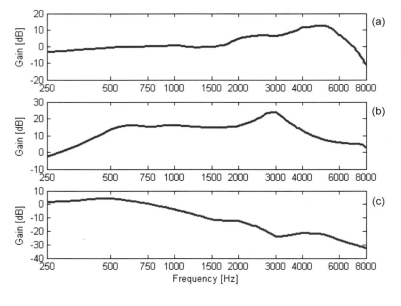

Figure 4–3   Transfer functions: **(a)** on the microphone side, **(b)** on the receiver side, and **(c)** on the parallel path.

receiver has a resonance peak of more than 20 dB at 3 kHz.

The vent mostly impacts the transfer function at low frequencies. **Figure 4–3b** shows how the gain decreases at frequencies below 500 Hz. The curve holds for a vent with a diameter of 2 mm. A narrower vent attenuates less, but at the same time also makes the *occlusion effect* worse.

Transfer Function of the Parallel Path

Next, we will look at the parallel path in **Fig. 4–3c**. Sound also travels from the free field through the vent into the ear canal. Again, there are two effects:

1. The pinna
2. The vent

Here, using **Figure 4–1** as a reference, we see that sound waves with frequencies up to 500 Hz reach the ear canal about as well as if there was no obstruction due to the hearing aid.

Basic Gain

Figure 4–4 shows the resulting transfer function when the three foregoing factors operate together. As mentioned before, this *basic gain* is effective under the assumption that the electronic module neither amplifies nor attenuates at all frequencies.

In practice, the electronic module amplifies too. This is necessary to provide the suitable gain to compensate for the individual hearing loss. Based on audiological data, a fitting software establishes target gains and the audiologist modifies them as needed. To carry the desired amplification into effect, the fitting software needs to take the *basic gain* into account in such a way that the gain programmed in the electronic module and the *basic gain* of the instrument together meet the amplification target. To this end, the fitting software needs to be aware of the hearing aid configuration (i.e., correct microphone and receiver definition, vent diameter, etc.).

Insertion Loss

An open ear amplifies sound from the free field, as we have seen in the Effects on the Acoustic Signal – By the Outer Ear subsection. Inserting a hearing aid into the ear canal invalidates the open ear response. This effect is called the *insertion loss*. The *insertion loss* also occurs due to an earmold in the ear canal.

Insertion loss makes it necessary to look more closely at gain specifications. The *basic gain* refers to the difference in sound pressure level at the tympanic membrane and in free field; this is referred to as *in-situ gain*. For a hearing-impaired person, however, another gain measure

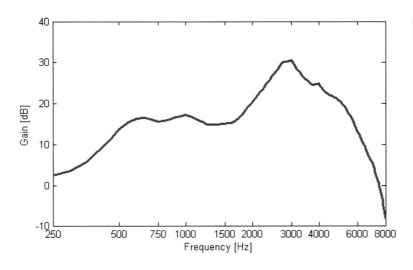

Figure 4–4   Basic gain of a hearing instrument.

is relevant: *insertion gain*. The relevant gain measure results from both *in-situ gain* and the lost open ear response:

$$\text{insertion gain} = \text{in-situ gain} - \text{open ear response} \quad \text{(Eq. 4-1)}$$

Example: **Figure 4–4** shows 31 dB *in-situ gain* at 3 kHz. Without a hearing aid, a hearing-impaired person already experiences 16 dB gain due to the open ear response. So, the hearing aid provides only 15 dB additional useful gain, and this is what *insertion gain* refers to.

◆ Linear Hearing Instrument

Linear hearing aids provide the same amplification for soft, average, and loud input signals. Checking their fitting flexibility thus requires another amplification target than the gain curves for WDRC that we looked at in the Digital Amplification Subsection in Chapter 3.

Figure 4–5 shows an appropriate amplification target, as established by the earlier NAL-RP fitting rationale (Byrne, 1986, 1990). NAL-RP specifies the amplification target in terms of

insertion gain. Conversion to in-situ gain is straightforward; rearranging the equation from the previous subsection yields:

$$\text{in-situ gain} = \text{insertion gain} + \text{open ear response} \quad \text{(Eq. 4-2)}$$

In **Fig. 4–5**, the vertical green lines illustrate how the in-situ gain target evolves from the prescribed insertion gain by adding the open ear response.

In the previous subsection, we also looked at a hearing aid's basic gain. Its shape across frequency grossly approximates the target correction for a sloping hearing loss. For our example, **Fig. 4–6** shows the remaining mismatch: 12 dB too much gain at 500 Hz and 6 dB too little gain at 1750 Hz.

Analog hearing instruments usually offered a few configurable filter stages to modify the basic gain. In our example, a simple high-pass filter reduces the mismatch at 500 Hz to 6 dB, but at the same time increases the mismatch at 1750 Hz to −8 dB. **Figure 4–6** also shows this corrected gain curve.

Using more filter stages might slightly improve the target match further. We will instead turn to the next processing scheme: broadband compression.

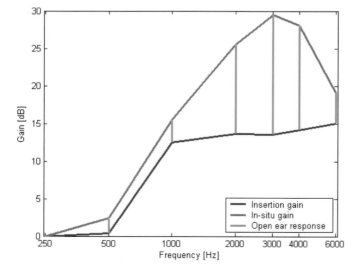

Figure 4–5   NAL-RP target gain for a sloping hearing loss.

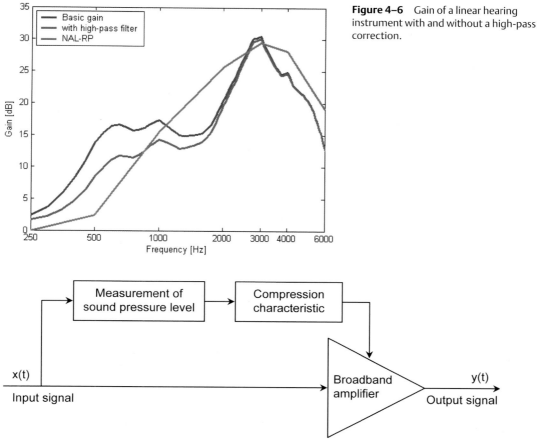

Figure 4–6   Gain of a linear hearing instrument with and without a high-pass correction.

Figure 4–7   Block diagram of a broadband compression system.

◆ Broadband Compression

Broadband compression starts from the gain curve of the linear hearing aid, as derived in the previous section. It additionally includes a broadband amplifier to vary the gain uniformly across frequency. **Figure 4–7** shows the block diagram.

The input signal x(t) goes to the *broadband amplifier* and also connects to the block *measurement of sound pressure level* on the upper signal path. This block continuously calculates the level of the input signal and passes the value on to the block *compression characteristic*. This second block continuously evaluates the amount of gain to apply and passes the value on to the *broadband amplifier*. The *broadband*

amplifier continuously provides the output signal y(t) while permanently adjusting its gain.

Figure 4–8 shows the gain curves that this simple processing scheme produces, together with the level-dependent NAL-NL1 amplification targets that we looked at in Chapter 3. As gain varies uniformly across frequency, the gain curves run more or less parallel to each other, with the exception of the low-frequency region below 750 Hz. At these frequencies the vent allows the sound from free field to pass directly into the ear canal. Direct sound therefore dominates when gain in the low frequencies gets below ~3 dB.

Broadband compression has a fundamental disadvantage. It lacks the flexibility to meet the amplification target in all frequency regions simultaneously. This is because the amplifica-

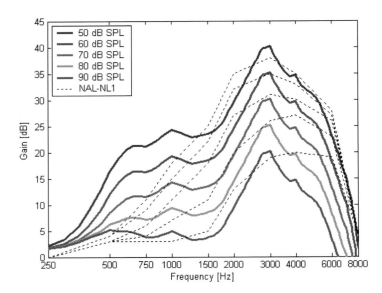

Figure 4–8　Target match with broadband compression.

tion targets do not run in parallel – in contrast to the gain curves. In our example, the target match is thus much better at 3 kHz than in the range between 500 Hz and 1 kHz.

The WDRC scheme in the next section improves the target match by splitting the input signal into separate frequency bands and processing these band signals separately. But before going on, let us review the commonly used compression diagrams:

◆ **Figure 4–9a** shows the compression characteristic

◆ **Figure 4–9b** illustrates the input–output characteristic

Table 4–2 details the average gain and output level for the input levels of 50, 60, 70, 80,

Table 4–2　Gain and Output Level for Different Input Levels

Input Level	Average Gain	Output Level
50 dB SPL	25 dB	75 dB SPL
60 dB SPL	20 dB	80 dB SPL
70 dB SPL	15 dB	85 dB SPL
80 dB SPL	10 dB	90 dB SPL
90 dB SPL	5 dB	95 dB SPL

SPL, sound pressure level.

and 90 dB SPL. This data determine the curves in **Fig. 4–9** as follows:

◆ For input levels up to 50 dB SPL, the hearing aid has an average gain of 25 dB; an input signal with 50 dB SPL therefore produces an output signal of 75 dB SPL.

◆ As the level of the input signal increases beyond 50 dB SPL, the hearing instrument reduces gain: at 90 dB SPL the gain is only 5 dB, giving an output signal of 95 dB SPL.

Although the input signal goes up from 50 dB SPL to 90 dB SPL, a 40 dB rise, the output signal only increases from 75 dB SPL to 95 dB SPL, a 20 dB rise. The following commonly used terms capture the compression characteristic:

◆ The *kneepoint* defines the level where compression sets in: 50 dB SPL in our example.

◆ The *compression ratio* indicates by how many dB the input signal must go up for the output signal to increase by 1 dB: in our example by 2 dB, therefore the compression ratio equals 2.

The idea of two-channel WDRC in the next section is to apply separate compression characteristics to the signals in two disjoint frequency bands. This allows for matching amplification targets better across all frequencies.

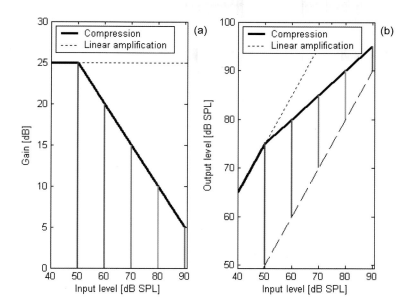

Figure 4–9 Characteristics of wide dynamic range compression: **(a)** Compression characteristic and **(b)** input–output characteristic.

◆ Two-channel Wide Dynamic Range Compression

Two-channel WDRC is based on the general principle of "divide and conquer." In our context, this means splitting the input signal into two band signals, a low-frequency signal and a high-frequency signal. The low-frequency signal contains the signal components with frequencies lower than a fixed cutoff frequency, and the high-frequency signal contains those signal components with higher frequencies. Using band signals makes it possible to apply different compression characteristics in different frequency regions, thereby getting closer to the targets.

In our example, a cutoff frequency of 1.5 kHz is the most suitable. This choice allows the application of different compression characteristics below and above 1.5 kHz, as **Fig. 4–10** shows. **Figure 4–10a** shows the compression characteristic for the low-frequency signal, and **Figure 4–10b** for the high-frequency signal.

Figure 4–11 shows the result: a better overall target match. Separate processing in two frequency bands removes the excessive gain that the broadband compression scheme showed in the frequency region below 1.5 kHz.

There is an interesting detail to mention at this point: applying separate gain in two frequency ranges should make the gain curves look like two steps of a staircase. So, why does **Fig. 4–11** show something different? Answer: the gain curves in **Fig. 4–11** depict the combination of electronic gain and basic gain; the electronic module on its own actually provides the step-shaped gain curves, as the colored lines in **Fig. 4–12** illustrate. The dashed black lines display the gain curves, when the electronic module includes the high-pass filter introduced with the linear hearing instrument in the Linear Hearing Instrument section.

So far, two-channel WDRC seems straightforward. Yet the block diagrams in **Fig. 4–13** and **Fig. 4–14** hold a surprise. They show two possible implementations. In both block diagrams, a low- and a high-pass filter split the input signal x(t) into band signals, separate amplifiers amplify the band signals and an adder combines the amplified band signals to form the output signal y(t). The block diagrams differ only in the quantity that adjusts each variable-gain amplifier. In **Fig. 4–13,** the levels of the two band signals drive the amplifiers. In **Fig. 4–14,** the level of the entire signal determines how much to amplify the two band signals.

What pops up here is the question regarding the number of independent compression channels. **Figure 4–13** depicts what is commonly referred to as two-channel WDRC, featuring

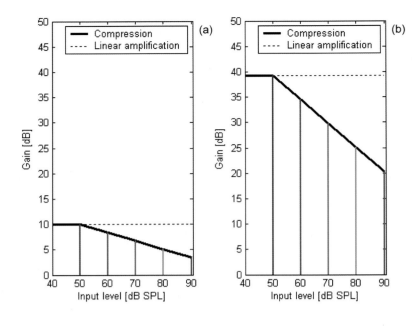

Figure 4–10 Compression characteristics in different frequency ranges: **(a)** low-frequency range and **(b)** high-frequency range.

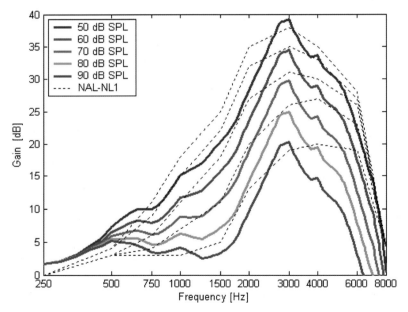

Figure 4–11 Target match with two-channel wide dynamic range compression.

two independent compression channels. The block diagram in **Fig. 4–14**, on the other hand, is rather designated as two-band WDRC. The concept of bands and channels is not well established; however, the terms are also used interchangeably and experts have different opinions about the required number of channels and bands (Mueller, 2000).

Two-channel WDRC originates from the idea of normalizing loudness independently in different frequency bands. It became common practice in analog instruments and, following

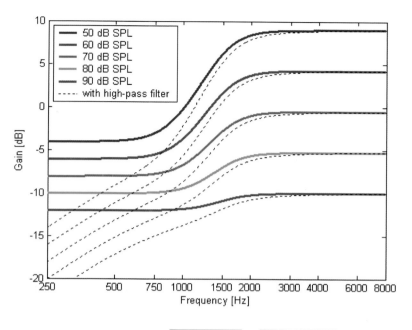

Figure 4–12 Two-channel wide dynamic range compression: gain provided by the electronic module.

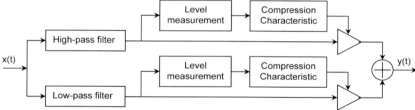

Figure 4–13 Block diagram of two-channel wide dynamic range compression.

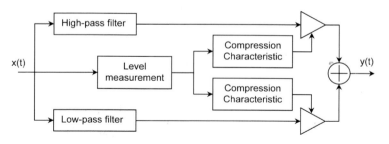

Figure 4–14 Block diagram of wide dynamic range compression in two bands.

technical advances, led to multichannel WDRC.

However, multiband WDRC is inherently better suited to matching amplification targets – of NAL-NL1 or any other fitting procedure. This happens by

◆ Defining the compression characteristics in separate frequency ranges – amplification targets in fact specify how much to amplify at different frequencies for different sound pressure levels of the input signal

◆ Applying these separate compression characteristics according to the sound pressure level of the input signal

With multichannel WDRC, matching amplification targets gets more complex. The problem lies in the actual gain deviating dynamically from the target gain, depending on the relative signal level in individual channels and on the speed of compression. As a result, the signal loses spectral contrast; in Chapter 6, we will look at how this effect originates.

Let us conclude by looking at two more aspects regarding channels and bands:

1. Commercial two-channel WDRC instruments may be comprised of multiple bands to provide better gain shaping capability. Example: the study (Schum & Pogash, 2003) mentioned in the previous chapter used a first-generation DSP instrument with seven bands that are assembled into two channels.

2. The belief in more and more compression channels has gradually decreased. Keidser and Grant (2001) report no significant difference in speech recognition for WDRC in one, two, or four channels; and no preference for either scheme for most subjects. Among those who preferred a scheme, some favored one channel and some two.

◆ Summary

This chapter started with the objectives of WDRC. The next section addressed the various effects that amplify or attenuate sound as it travels from the free field to the tympanic membrane. We then looked at three basic amplification strategies: a linear hearing aid, broadband compression, and two-channel WDRC. In each case the focus was on the flexibility that the instrument provides in fitting to the individual hearing loss.

References

Bentler, R. A., and Duve, M. R. (2000). Comparison of hearing aids over the 20th century. Ear & Hearing, 21(6), 625–39.

Byrne, D., and Dillon, H. (1986). The national acoustics laboratories' (NAL) new procedure for selecting gain and frequency response of a hearing aid. Ear & Hearing, 7(4), 257–265.

Byrne, D., Parkinson, A., and Newall, P. (1990). Hearing aid gain and frequency response requirements for the severely/profoundly hearing impaired. Ear & Hearing, 11(1), 40-49.

Dillon H. (1999). NAL-NL1: A new prescriptive fitting procedure for non-linear hearing aids. The Hearing Journal, 52(4), 10–16.

———. (2001). Hearing aids. New York: Thieme Medical Publishers.

Hansen, M. (2002). Effects of multi-channel compression time constants on subjectively perceived sound quality and speech intelligibility. Ear & Hearing, 23(4), 369–380.

Humes, L. E., Christensen, L., Thomas, T., Bess, F. H., Hedley-Williams, A., Bentler, R. (1999). A comparison of the aided performance and benefit provided by a linear and a two-channel wide dynamic range compression hearing aid. Journal of Speech, Language, and Hearing Research, 42(1), 65–79.

Keidser, G., Dillon, H., and Brewer, S. (1999). Using the NAL-NL1 prescriptive procedure with advanced hearing instruments. The Hearing Review, 6(11), 8–20.

Keidser, G., and Grant, F. (2001). The preferred number of channels (one, two, or four) in NAL-NL1 prescribed wide dynamic range compression (WDRC) devices. Ear & Hearing, 22(6), 516–527.

———. (2003). Loudness normalization or speech intelligibility maximization? Differences in clinical goals, issues, and preferences. The Hearing Review, 10(1): 14–25.

Larson, V. D., Williams, D. W., Henderson, W. G., Luethke, L. E., Beck, L. B., Noffsinger, D., et al. (2000). Efficacy of 3 commonly used hearing aid circuits: A crossover trial. NIDCD/VA Hearing Aid Clinical Trial Group. Journal of the American Medical Association, 284(11), 1806–1813.

Marriage, J. E., and Moore, B. C. (2003). New speech tests reveal benefit of wide-dynamic-range, fast-acting compression for consonant discrimination in children with moderate-to-profound hearing loss. International Journal of Audiology, 42(7), 418–425.

Mueller, H. G. (2000). What's the digital difference when it comes to patient benefit? The Hearing Journal, 53(3), 23–32.

Schum, D. J., and Pogash, R. R. (2003). Blinded comparison of three levels of hearing aid technology. The Hearing Review, 10(1), 40–43, 64–65.

Valente, M., and Van Vliet, D. (1997). The independent hearing aid fitting forum (IHAFF) protocol. Trends in Amplification, 2(1), 6–35.

Venema T. (2006). Compression for clinicians (2nd ed.). Clifton Park, NY: Thomson Delmar Learning.

Part II

Signal Processing in Digital Hearing Aids

5

Static Behavior of Digital Wide Dynamic Range Compression

In this chapter, the discussion of fitting flexibility is continued, now focusing on digital technology. At some points it will be necessary to understand the digital signal. The sections in this chapter thus deal with

1. *The digital signal*: How does it represent the analog waveform of an acoustic signal?

2. *Wide dynamic range compression (WDRC) with transformation into the frequency domain*: transforms the input signal into a spectrum in the frequency domain, changes the spectrum, and transforms it back into the output signal in the time domain

3. *WDRC with a filter bank*: uses a filter bank to split the input signal into separate band signals, compresses the band signals and recombines them to form a single output signal

4. *WDRC with a controllable filter*: uses a controllable filter to amplify the input signal in both a frequency- and level-dependent way, thus producing the output signal

In Chapter 3, I addressed the question of the digital advantage, including all additional features that digital hearing aids provide. Here the question is how digital WDRC compares to analog WDRC. Studies usually deny an advantage when exploring comparable digital and analog instruments (Walden et al, 2000; Bille et al, 1999; Ricketts & Dhar, 1999), or find just a slight performance advantage (Ringdahl et al, 2000). This is no surprise. There is no reason why the two technologies should produce different results given that they implement the same processing schemes.

As we will see in this chapter, digital WDRC, however, offers much higher fitting flexibility. This raises new questions: Is this improvement just overkill? Or do clinicians perhaps not adequately use it in practice (Smriga, 2004)? Audiologists should be aware that fitting software usually shows more insertion gain in the high frequencies than the hearing aids actually produce (Hawkins & Cook, 2003). Nonetheless, only about a third of the audiologists use probe-microphones routinely, and only 30% routinely conduct aided speech measures (Mueller, 2003).

As mentioned before, the focus here is on looking at how digital signal processing works in today's hearing instruments, regardless of how much user benefit each improvement provides on its own. For a more detailed discussion, see Venema (2006) and Dillon (2001).

◆ The Digital Signal

At the start of the 1990s, it became apparent that the transformation from analog to digital technology was about to hit the hearing aid industry. A decade earlier, the compact disc (CD) had replaced the long-playing (LP) record. Sound pressure had been recorded in a continuous profile along a groove on an LP. In the case of a CD, because it only stores numbers, sound pressure is recorded at short, regular time intervals in a number series. Every number is coded with sufficient resolution to provide accurate sound reproduction with a dynamic range of 90 dB.

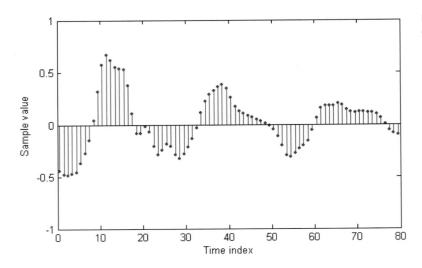

Figure 5–1   Example of a digital signal.

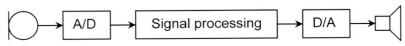

Figure 5–2   Additional signal converters in a digital hearing instrument.

Figure 5–1 depicts a digital signal, or more precisely, a sampled signal, where the sample values record the signal waveform at discrete intervals. This signal representation features regular vertical lines in the form of "pins." The heads of the pins follow the sound pressure of an acoustic signal over 5 ms. The lengths of the pins corresponds to the value of the sound pressure at each time point.

There is a time index along the x-axis, numbering the individual sample values sequentially. And a normalized number format is usual for the y-axis, with values between -1 and $+1$.

The diagram contains 80 sample values in the 5-ms segment; this corresponds to a sampling rate of 16 kHz (i.e., 16,000 samples per second). A sampling rate of 16 to 20 kHz is standard for hearing instruments. Then the instrument can cope with acoustic signals that have a bandwidth of up to 8 or 10 kHz, respectively. The digital signals on CDs feature a sampling rate of 44.1 kHz and thus represent acoustic signals with a bandwidth of 22.05 kHz.

As **Figure 5–2** shows, a digital hearing aid requires special signal converters: an analog-to-digital converter (A/D) and a digital-to-analog converter (D/A). Signal processing from microphone to receiver is composed of these three steps:

1. The A/D converter transforms the continuous microphone signal into a series of numbers.

2. A digital integrated circuit processes the input series of numbers to create the output signal – as another series of numbers.

3. The D/A converter transforms the output series of numbers back into a continuous signal for the receiver to emit.

This short review of the digital signal will facilitate the reader's understanding of the processing schemes given in the next three sections. For a more detailed discussion, see Decker and Carrell (2004).

◆ Wide Dynamic Range Compression with Transformation into the Frequency Domain

Hearing aids, thanks to digital technology, now use completely new methods to process an acoustic signal. The *discrete Fourier transform* is a

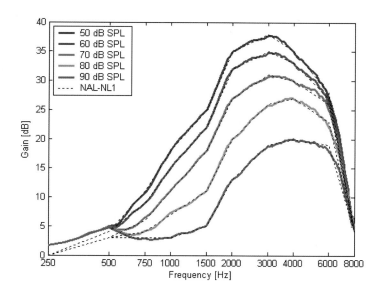

Figure 5–3   Target match using wide dynamic range compression with a transformation into the frequency domain.

typical example. Using this transformation, the hearing aid is able to calculate the spectrum of a sampled signal. The result is another series of numbers: samples of the spectrum at regular intervals along the frequency-axis. In Chapter 11, we will examine in detail how this transformation works; here the focus is on the fitting flexibility that the processing scheme provides.

Digital signal processing also offers the opposite process: the *inverse discrete Fourier transform*. Given the sample values of a spectrum, the inverse Fourier transform creates the corresponding sample values of a signal segment along the time axis.

In relation to hearing aid technology, the discrete Fourier transform is interesting because it allows processing the acoustic signal directly in the frequency domain. Once the spectrum samples are calculated, it is possible to amplify each of them by the exact amount of gain desired at each frequency. In this process, the overall shaping of the gain curve gets better and better, the closer the spectrum samples lie to one another along the frequency axis.

Sample values every 125 Hz produce a perfect target match, as **Fig. 5–3** shows. To appreciate this result, it is necessary to recall the gain curves from the previous chapter: the target match of broadband compression in **Fig. 4–8** or of two-channel WDRC in **Fig. 4–11**. Those gain curves still look somewhat similar to the basic

gain derived in Chapter 4's subsection, Effects on the Acoustic Signal by an Instrument in the Ear Canal, and depicted in **Fig. 4–4**. This is so because of the limited means that the analog processing schemes offer to modify the basic gain. Consequently, effects that determine the basic gain remain visible to some extent, especially the resonance peak of the receiver.

With the Fourier transform the situation is completely different; its capability to shape the gain curve is enormous. As **Fig. 5–3** shows, this technique allows compensating for all peaks and troughs in the basic gain, except for the frequency region below 500 Hz, where direct sound through the vent dominates.

One thing needs to be clarified at this point: seeking a perfect target match might erroneously be understood as overvaluing the significance of prescribed target gain. The idea here is quite different. The better a processing scheme matches the amplification targets, the more closely it will also follow each modification in the subsequent fine-tuning process. The particular target gain curves used here just serve as a realistic example; they make it possible to compare the fitting flexibility of various processing techniques.

WDRC with transformation into the frequency domain also has a minor disadvantage. When aiming at a perfect target match, the processing scheme is likely to produce an objectionable processing delay (Agnew & Thornton, 2000). Hearing aid wearers usually dislike their own voice when the hearing instrument delays the sound by more than 10 ms. Reducing the frequency resolution, spectrum samples every 250 Hz or 500 Hz, for example, shortens the processing delay and thus diminishes the disturbing effect to barely noticeable. So, the Fourier transform is a valuable technique. But alternative implementations also have their merits, as we will see in the sections ahead.

◆ Wide Dynamic Range Compression with a Filter Bank

Many digital signal-processing strategies closely parallel their old analog counterparts. Some processing schemes, for instance, split the input signal into separate frequency bands, with digital filters where analog filters were used earlier. In Chapter 12, I will show by means of a sample calculation how digital filters split a signal into two frequency bands.

Even when mirroring the original approach, digital signal processing occasionally opens up new possibilities. For instance, by using a *filter bank* the input signal is split simultaneously

into multiple band signals; thus, two-channel WDRC becomes *multichannel* WDRC.

In this section, we will look at the fitting flexibility of a processing scheme that splits the input signal into eight frequency bands. **Figure 5–4** shows the target match. Two aspects stand out in this diagram:

1. The gain curves show a distinct peak at 3 kHz. This is because of the limited means that the eight-band approach provides for modifying the basic gain. Hence the resonance peak of the receiver remains visible – in marked contrast to the Fourier transform approach described in the previous section.

    It should also be noted that using bandpass filters with little overlap may even make matters worse. In **Fig. 5–4**, the gain curves for the high input levels show an additional peak at 5 kHz; this happens because applying different gains in different frequency bands may produce a staircase-shaped gain curve; **Fig. 5–5** shows how the electronic module amplifies on its own. The electronic gain combines with the slope of the receiver resonance and occasionally produces additional peaks.

2. The gain curves for input levels of 60, 70, and 80 dB SPL deviate more from the amplification

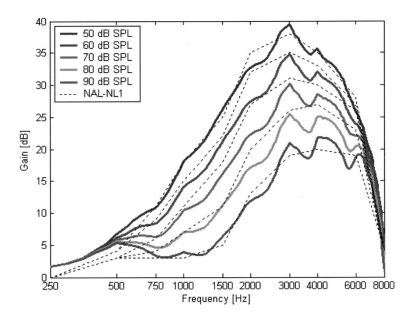

Figure 5–4 Target match using eight-channel wide dynamic range compression and conventional compression characteristics.

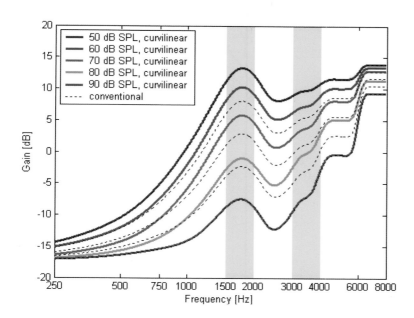

Figure 5–5 Eight-channel wide dynamic range compression: gain provided by the electronic module.

targets than those for 50 and 90 dB SPL. This effect is due to conventional compression characteristics that have a kneepoint and a fixed compression ratio, as introduced with broadband compression in Chapter 4.

Digital hearing aids usually apply more flexible *curvilinear* characteristics. **Figure 5–6** illustrates the difference for the input–output characteristics in two frequency bands: **Fig. 5–6a** in the frequency range from 1.5 to 2 kHz, and **Fig. 5–6b** from 3 to 4 kHz.

The *curvilinear* characteristics impact the gain curves; the dashed black lines in **Fig. 5–5** show the gain curves for conventional characteristics, and the solid colored curves the ones for the curvilinear characteristics. The yellow shaded areas mark the two frequency ranges that we considered more closely: 1.5 to 2 kHz and 3 to 4 kHz.

Combining electronic gain and basic gain produces the gain curves that **Fig. 5–7** displays. The *curvilinear* characteristics improve the target match at the intermediate input levels of 60, 70, and 80 dB SPL. The peaks and troughs across frequency remain, however; the curvilinear characteristics have no impact on this.

The *filter bank* approach holds further potential. It is usually straightforward to extend the processing scheme in such a way that it splits the input signal into more

frequency bands. This extension gradually enhances the capability in gain shaping until it approaches that of the Fourier transform in the previous section.

The processing delay of WDRC with a filter bank increases with the number of band signals that the filter bank generates; it is possible, however, to keep it below 3 ms, and thus remains imperceptible to the hearing aid user (Agnew & Thornton, 2000).

Therefore, WDRC with a filter bank is another valuable option.

◆ Wide Dynamic Range Compression with a Controllable Filter

WDRC with the Fourier transform or with a filter bank both take the acoustic signal apart in somewhat rigid, arbitrary – and altogether unnecessary – ways:

◆ The *discrete Fourier transform* splits the signal into consecutive segments of equal length.

◆ The *filter bank* cuts it into a fixed number of frequency bands with fixed bandwidths.

Controllable filters are different: they produce continuous gain functions and process the

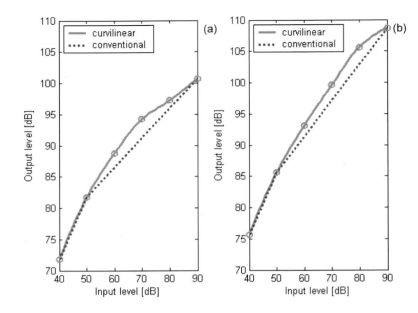

Figure 5–6   Input–output characteristics at different frequencies: **(a)** in the range 1.5 to 2 kHz and **(b)** in the range 3 to 4 kHz.

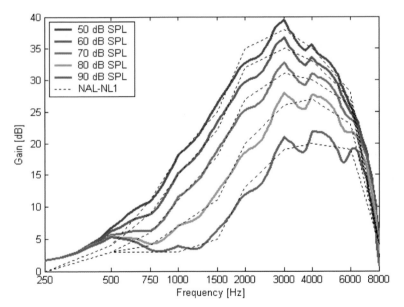

Figure 5–7   Target match using eight-channel wide dynamic range compression with curvilinear characteristics.

signal continuously, without splitting it in any fixed way.

Figure 5–8 and **Fig. 5–9** show two block diagrams containing controllable filters. In both diagrams there are two parallel signal paths: a main path and a secondary path. Passing along the main path, the input signal first encounters a *synchronization* block. This *synchronization*

ensures that the signal progression in both paths remains in step. We will look more closely at what this means when dealing with *signal overshoot* in Chapter 6.

Next, the signal reaches a *controllable filter*. It amplifies the signal in a frequency- and level-dependent way, such that the hearing aid permanently approaches the amplification targets

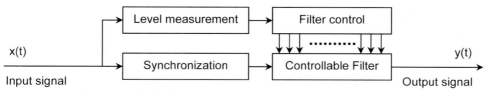

Figure 5–8   Block diagram of wide dynamic range compression with a controllable lattice filter.

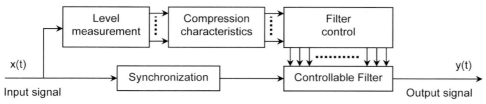

Figure 5–9   Block diagram of wide dynamic range compression with a controllable finite impulse response filter.

as closely as possible. This task involves the hardest challenge with these processing schemes: modifying the gain curve of the *controllable filter* on the fly, while the sound pressure level of the input signal continuously changes.

Filter design is already considered a demanding chore without the additional condition to perform it in real-time. Regarding the system in **Fig. 5–8**, the filter update algorithm exceeds the scope of this book; for details, see Schaub and Leber (2002). For the system depicted in **Fig. 5–9**, however, I will elaborate on the system using a simplified model in Chapter 12; for more detail, see Schaub (2004).

In both block diagrams, the *filter control* block performs the magic of continuously updating the filter gain curve. To this end, the *filter control* continuously adjusts parameters in the *controllable filter*; this is what the many parallel arrows from the *filter control* to the *controllable filter* indicate in the block diagrams.

In **Fig. 5–8**, the *filter control* operates directly from the input level that the *level measurement* block calculates. In **Fig. 5–9**, however, there is an additional *compression characteristics* block between *level measurement* and *filter control*. The *compression characteristics* here serve the same purpose as described in the previous chapter: they specify how much to amplify for any given input level. The system given in

Fig. 5–9 is configurable and makes it possible to vary the number of frequency bands with separate compression characteristics.

In the two block diagrams, there are two different types of *controllable filters*: a *lattice filter* in **Fig. 5–8**, and an *FIR filter* in **Fig. 5–9**. The term *lattice filter* derives from the structure that shows up when sketching the signal flow that this type of filter possesses. The acronym *FIR*, on the other hand, stands for *finite impulse response*. An isolated pulsed input signal causes this type of filter to produce an output signal that quickly dies away. For an introduction to both filter types, see Padmanabhan et al (2001).

Let us now return to the focus of this chapter and check the fitting flexibility that these processing schemes provide.

Controllable Lattice Filter

The first step in using the controllable lattice filter consists of calculating filter parameters for each of a limited number of input signal levels. The fitting software performs this step according to the individual hearing loss and allows for the basic gain of the instrument. **Figure 5–10** shows the result for input levels of 50, 60, 70, 80, and 90 dB SPL. These gain curves are continuous, with no sign of a staircase-shape. Combining this electronic gain with the basic gain of the hearing instrument produces the gain curves

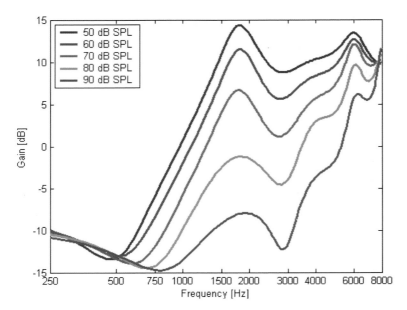

Figure 5–10   Wide dynamic range compression with a controllable lattice filter: gain provided by the electronic module.

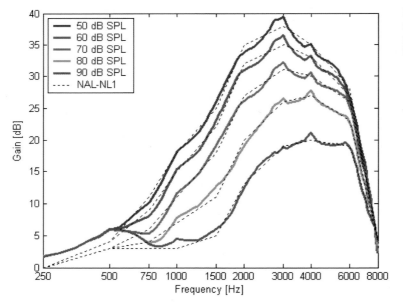

Figure 5–11   Target match using wide dynamic range compression with a controllable lattice filter.

that **Fig. 5–11** shows. The target match is close to that of the Fourier transform approach described in a previous section. The approach here, however, produces a processing delay of 1 to 1.5 ms only – short enough to remain imperceptible to the hearing aid user (Agnew & Thornton, 2000).

As mentioned before, the main challenge with the controllable filter is to modify its gain curve on the fly. **Figure 5–12** illustrates how this works. The sound pressure level of the input signal rarely matches exactly 50, 60, 70, 80, or 90 dB SPL. For all other levels, the *filter control* block calculates interpolated filter

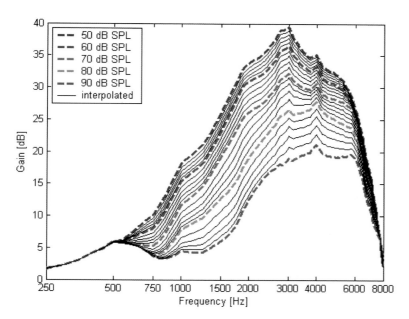

Figure 5–12   Interpolated gain curves with a controllable lattice filter.

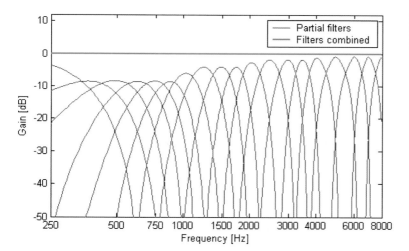

Figure 5–13   Partial transfer functions of a controllable finite impulse response filter.

parameters. To this end, the precalculated filter parameters serve as starting values; **Fig. 5–12** shows their corresponding gain curves as colored dashed lines. And the black solid lines show interpolated gain curves for input levels 2 dB apart from each other. In practice, interpolation produces different gain curves for input levels that differ only by a fraction of 1 dB.

WDRC with a controllable lattice filter is another valuable option. Its design avoids splitting the input signal into bands or channels. Hence, the term ChannelFree evolved to designate this processing scheme. A hearing instrument using this technique took part in a test on sound quality (Dillon et al, 2003): hearing-impaired listeners gave it the highest average scores for male and female voices as well as for piano music.

Controllable Finite Impulse Response Filter

The controllable FIR filter emanates from a set of FIR band-pass filters, as **Fig. 5–13** shows. If each band-pass filter amplifies as shown, then

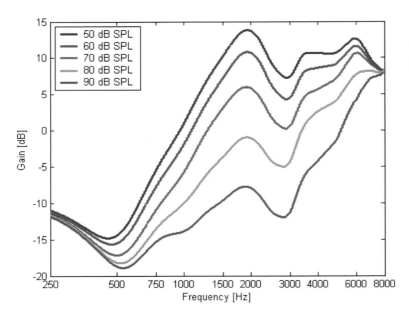

Figure 5–14   Wide dynamic range compression with a controllable finite impulse response filter: gain provided by the electronic module.

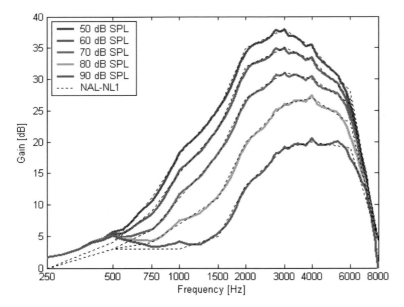

Figure 5–15   Target match using wide dynamic range compression with a controllable finite impulse response filter.

their combined action produces 0 dB gain across frequency. To achieve a particular gain curve, some of the band-pass filters need to amplify more, and others less.

Although **Fig. 5–13** is reminiscent of a filter bank, the individual filters here are combined differently. Recall that the filter bank splits the input signal into band signals and processes the signal parts separately. The controllable FIR

filter takes another approach: it combines the different filters into one single filter and processes the input signal as a whole.

Figure 5–14 shows the gain curves of the controllable FIR filter for input levels of 50, 60, 70, 80 and 90 dB SPL. Combining this electronic gain with the basic gain of the instrument produces the gain curves that **Fig. 5–15** shows. The target match is close to that of the

Fourier transform approach; the system here, however, produces a processing delay of 2.4 ms only – short enough to remain imperceptible to the hearing aid user (Agnew & Thornton, 2000).

The filter update mechanism of the controllable FIR filter works differently from that of the controllable lattice filter, as we shall see in Chapter 12 starting from a simplified model.

Therefore, WDRC with a controllable FIR filter is still another valuable option.

◆ Summary

This chapter started with a short review of the characteristics of digital signals. The next three sections presented valuable options for performing WDRC with digital technology: WDRC with transformation into frequency domain, with a filter bank, and with controllable filters. In conclusion, the digital technology provides higher fitting flexibility than does analog technology. This is essential for matching prescribed targets and for subsequent changes to the amplification in fine-tuning sessions.

References

Agnew, J., and Thornton J. M. (2000). Just noticeable and objectionable group delays in digital hearing aids. Journal of the American Academy of Audiology, 11(6), 330–336.

Bille, M., Jensen, A. M., Kjaerbol, E., Vesterager, V., Sibelle, P., and Nielsen, H. (1999). Clinical study of a digital vs. an analogue hearing aid. Scandinavian Audiology, 28(2), 127–135.

Decker, T. N., and Carell, T. D. (2004). Instrumentation: An introduction for students in the speech and hearing sciences. Mahwah, NJ: Lawrence Erlbaum Associates.

Dillon, H. (2001). Hearing aids. New York: Thieme Medical Publishers.

Dillon, H., Keidser, G., O'Brien, A., and Silberstein, H. (2003). Sound quality comparisons of advanced hearing aids. The Hearing Journal, 56(4), 30–40.

Hawkins, D. B., and Cook, J. A. (2003). Hearing aid software predictive gain values: How accurate are they? The Hearing Journal, 56(7), 26–34.

Mueller, H. G. (2003). Fitting test protocols are "more honored in the breach than the observance." The Hearing Journal, 56(10), 19–26.

Padmanabhan, K., Ananthi, S., and Vijayarajeswaran, R. (2003). A practical approach to digital signal processing. New Delhi, India: New Age International.

Ricketts, T., and Dhar, S. (1999). Comparison of performance across three directional hearing aids. Journal of the American Academy of Audiology, 10(4), 180–189.

Ringdahl, A., Magnusson, L., Edberg, P., and Thelin, L. (2000). Clinical evaluation of a digital power hearing instrument. The Hearing Review, 7(3), 59–64.

Schaub, A., and Leber, R. (2002). Loudness-controlled processing of acoustic signals. United States Patent, US 6,370,255 B1, Apr. 9.

Schaub, A. (2004). Signal processing in a hearing aid. United States Patent Application Publication, Pub. No. US 2004/0175011 A1, Sept. 9.

Smriga, D.J. (2004). How to measure and demonstrate four key digital hearing aid performance features. The Hearing Review, 11(11), 30–38.

Venema T. (2006). Compression for clinicians (2nd ed.). New York: Thieme Medical Publishers.

Walden, B. E., Surr, R. K., Cord, M. T., Edwards, B., and Olson, L. (2000). Comparison of benefits provided by different hearing aid technologies. Journal of the American Academy of Audiology, 11(10), 540–560.

6

Temporal Behavior of Digital Wide Dynamic Range Compression

The temporal behavior of wide dynamic range compression (WDRC) involves the speed at which a hearing aid adjusts gain when the sound pressure level of the input signal changes. There are two aspects of this behavior.

1. How fast the instrument reduces the gain, when the sound pressure level increases—commonly referred to as *attack time*

2. How fast the instrument increases the amplification when the sound pressure level goes down—commonly referred to as *release time*

The question, which deals with one of the basic objectives of WDRC, is whether to implement a fast-acting system or a slow automatic volume control.

Attack and *release times* are among the most controversial topics. Mueller (2000) interviewed experts from seven hearing aid manufacturers. They recommended compression speed from "really fast" to "really slow," *release time* from 20 ms to 20 s. Why this extreme disparity? Sound pressure level is a definite, physical quantity; the standard (IEC, 2002) specifies how to measure it. The standard is about sound level meters, however, and specifies 125 ms as a "fast" time constant. An *attack time* of 125 milliseconds is all right for a measurement instrument; however, for a hearing aid it is far too long. In case of a burst noise, a hearing aid must reduce amplification much faster and thereby avoid emitting too loud a sound.

Hence hearing aid manufacturers had to find their own way in coping with the varying signal level in speech. Consequently, they came up with different strategies. The longer the release

time, the more slowly a WDRC system behaves. It still has the potential to provide uniform speech recognition across various levels, from soft speech to shouted speech, as reported by Jenstad et al (1999). To compensate for a damaged cochlea, the WDRC should be fast, however (Edwards, 2001). The aim is to increase the consonant recognition in ongoing speech (Kennedy et al, 1998; Smith & Levitt, 2000); the approach occasionally results in some benefit (Marriage & Moore, 2003).

The faster a WDRC system should work, the more care it takes to avoid distortions and signal degradation. One particular strategy accomplishes virtually instantaneous WDRC. However, let us first address what actually determines the temporal behavior.

In Chapter 4, we looked at the block diagram of a two-channel WDRC system. Both compression channels in **Fig. 4–13** contained three blocks: a *level measurement* block, a *compression characteristic* block, and a *variable-gain amplifier*. They perform these three continuous actions:

1. Measure the input level

2. Translate the input level into the desired gain, i.e., apply the compression characteristic

3. Amplify the signal while permanently adjusting the gain

Actions 2 and 3 happen with virtually no delay. Only action 1—level measurement—takes time and actually determines the temporal behavior of a WDRC system.

The sections in this chapter will thus address

1. *Measuring the sound pressure level*: What are the basics of level measurement? And what

does it take to acquire accurate and virtually instantaneous measurement values?

2. *Undesired side effects*: loss of spectral contrast and signal overshoot. When do these effects occur and how can they be diminished?

For further discussion on topics related to the temporal behavior of WRCD, see Venema (2006) or Dillon (2001).

◆ Measuring the Sound Pressure Level

Measuring the sound pressure level relies on observing sound pressure oscillations over a certain period. The length of this time interval determines whether a system behaves as a slow automatic volume control or performs fast-acting WDRC. This time interval is also known as the *observation window.*

A short observation window means that the measurement value changes quickly. As a result, the WDRC system changes its amplification quickly too. A long observation window, on the other hand, produces a slowly changing average measurement. Consequently, the WDRC system amplifies by almost the same amount over a long time. Next, we will look at the observation window and see how the notion of a *time constant* relates to it.

Then we will consider different measurement methods and the results they record. Using clearly defined test signals allows us to predict the results that they should produce, thus revealing any shortcomings. Subsequently, we will examine how the different methods process speech signals.

The Observation Window

As discussed in Chapter 5, there are different approaches to digital WDRC: using a transformation into the frequency domain, a filter bank, or controllable filters. There is also a variety of measurement procedures for recording the input sound-pressure level, which suit the various approaches differently. For example, if a hearing aid processes the input signal in consecutive segments, as when transforming it into the frequency domain, these segments form natural observation windows for the level measurement. The hearing aid determines a new measurement value in each segment, and also establishes how much gain to apply to the signal components at the different frequencies. In this case, an observation window typically lasts for 10 ms.

Calculating the sound pressure level in short consecutive segments has both an advantage and a disadvantage. The advantage is that the measurement value tracks the short-term sound pressure level of consecutive phonemes in speech because the segment is shorter than the phonemes. For this reason, the *segmental value* will serve the purpose of a reference value when it comes to measuring the sound pressure level of speech signals in a following subsection.

The disadvantage is that the *segmental value* sometimes changes in large steps from one segment to the next; we will see an example when measuring the level of speech signals later in this chapter. The size of the step depends on the waveform of the signal. Calculating the sound pressure level of *overlapping segments* usually reduces the effect. In this case, a new value is calculated every 5 ms, while each segment is still 10 ms long. In the sections ahead, we will actually use the *segmental value* of *overlapping segments*, as it preserves the advantage of tracking the short-term sound pressure levels.

The observation window is quite different in WDRC systems that use a filter bank or a controllable filter. These systems involve ongoing gain adjustments using small steps, from one sample to the next. The continuous adjustment, however, entails recording a new level value for every sampling interval, determining the gain from it, and applying the gain to the signal. In Chapter 13, we will look at the calculations that digital signal processing methods use to achieve continuous level measurements. The main novelty is the use of a *sliding observation window*, as marked in red in **Fig. 6–1**. All three diagrams in the figure contain the same 300 ms extract taken from the word "understand," which we saw in Chapter 1.

Figure 6–1a shows a short observation window that has reached the time of 490 ms, as the vertical red boundary line indicates. The other two boundary lines define the window length. The farther apart they are from one another at a given time, the more the sound

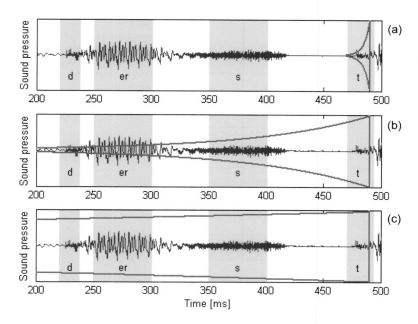

Figure 6–1 Observation window for different time constants: **(a)** 5 ms, **(b)** 100 ms, and **(c)** 1 s.

pressure from that point contributes to the measurement value, and the closer together they are, the less the sound pressure contributes. Therefore, the newest sample value contributes the most, and earlier samples contribute less the farther back in time they lie. With each new sample, the observation window slides one sampling interval further along.

In the example from **Fig. 6–1a,** the level measurement at time 490 ms is only based on the sound pressure of the phoneme /t/. **Figures 6–1b** and **6–1c,** on the other hand, have longer observation windows. Both have also reached 490 ms. In **Fig. 6–1b,** the sound pressure over 300 ms contributes to the level measurement, although the sample values at the start of the segment only have a minimal effect. The level measurement in **Fig. 6–1c** is based on the sound pressure across multiple syllables, even multiple preceding words. All sample values in the segment shown contribute strongly to the measurement.

It is usual to characterize the length of the observation window by a quantity known as a *time constant.* It defines the time taken for the red boundary curve to fall to around a third—more precisely to $e^{-1} \cong 37\%$. Time constants in **Figs. 6–1a—6–1c** are 5 ms, 100 ms, and 1 s, respectively.

The example of the stop consonant /t/ makes it clear: only a short time constant is suitable for measuring the sound pressure level separately for consecutive phonemes. Longer time constants have the effect that the measurement values are always based on multiple phonemes, sometimes multiple syllables, or even entire words.

Level Measurement of Test Signals

At first glance, it looks as if the acquisition of a fast measurement value only depends on choosing a short enough time constant for the level measurement. This is, however, a fallacy. A short time constant proves itself for simple test signals, such as the sinusoidal test signal from the standard (IEC, 1983); nevertheless, if the time constant is too short for real signals, it can lead to damaging measurement errors, as we will see shortly.

It is easy to avoid such measurement errors by using longer time constants. This, in turn, has its own risk. When the sound pressure level rises quickly, the level measurement drags behind, so the hearing aid amplifies the signal by too much for a while, causing the output signal to overshoot. For this reason, a measurement procedure using two different time constants is common

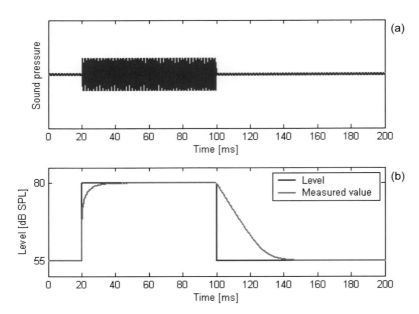

Figure 6–2 Level measurement using a short time constant: **(a)** waveform of a sinusoidal test signal and **(b)** sound pressure level and measurement value.

practice; one is used when the level goes up, and the other when it goes down. This method is known as *level measurement with asymmetric time constants.* Its disadvantages are that it only records a slowly changing measurement value and introduces a new measurement error. To acquire an accurate and virtually instantaneous level value thus requires yet another measurement procedure.

We will next determine

- How a short time constant correctly captures the sound pressure level of a sinusoidal test signal

- What measurement errors occur when using the same method for processing a pulsed test signal

- How the method of asymmetric time constants avoids these errors, but only records a slowly changing measurement value and even introduces a new error

- How to measure an accurate and virtually instantaneous level value instead

Level Measurement with Short Time Constants

The standard (IEC, 1983) describes guidelines for testing hearing aids that feature automatic gain control. **Figure 6–2a** shows the test signal that the standard proposes: a sinusoidal signal

with a frequency of 1600 Hz, and a sound pressure level that steps up from 55 to 80 dB SPL and then back to 55 dB SPL. The 80-ms-long signal segment at 80 dB SPL contains 128 oscillations; they are so close together that the signal appears as a solid block in the diagram.

Figure 6–2b shows the sound pressure level and the measured value obtained from a measurement with a time constant of 5 ms. The measurement value mostly matches the sound pressure level, apart from the time periods immediately following a level change; then the measurement takes time to settle to the new value.

What effect does a 5-ms time constant have on the measured value?

- For the jump from 55 to 80 dB SPL, the measured value increases to 78 dB SPL within 5 ms, getting to within 2 dB of the sound pressure level

- For the jump from 80 dB back down to 55 dB SPL, the measured value decreases by 4 dB during the first 5 ms; and it takes nearly six times as long, around 30 ms, for the measured value to get to within 2 dB of the true sound pressure level

This observation may be confusing, and begs the question: Are there two different time constants here? But it is not the case. This temporal behavior happens because measuring according to the norm (IEC, 2002) requires applying the observation window to squared sound pressure values and subsequently converting the result to a dB scale. We will look at this more closely in Chapter 13; here a short calculation will suffice to see how the effect comes about.

The basics given in Chapter 1 established the relation between sound pressure and sound pressure level:

$$L = 10 \cdot \log_{10}(p^2/p_0^2) = 20 \cdot \log_{10}(p/p_0) \quad \text{(Eq. 6-1)}$$

L gives the level in dB SPL, p the sound pressure in Pa, and the reference pressure p_0 is 20 μPa.

The formula can be rearranged to form:

$$p = 10^{L/20} \cdot p_0 \quad \text{(Eq. 6-2)}$$

Applying the sound pressure levels 55 and 80 dB SPL to this formula yields the sound pressures, and their squared values:

$$55 \text{ dB SPL} \rightarrow 11.25 \text{ mPa} \rightarrow 126 \text{ mPa}^2,$$
$$80 \text{ dB SPL} \rightarrow 200 \text{ mPa} \rightarrow 40{,}000 \text{ mPa}^2.$$

In our example, the square of the sound pressure jumps up by 39,874 mPa². Within the length of one time constant following a level jump, the measured value approaches the new value by around 37% of the height of the step—in this case by 14,669 mPa². Therefore, the square of the sound pressure reaches 25,331 mPa² (=40,000 mPa² − 14,669 mPa²) one time constant after the jump-up, and 14,795 mPa² (=126 mPa² + 14,669 mPa²) one time constant after the step-down. These values correspond to the following sound pressure levels:

$$25{,}331 \text{ mPa}^2 \rightarrow 159 \text{ mPa} \rightarrow 78 \text{ dB SPL},$$
$$14{,}795 \text{ mPa}^2 \rightarrow 122 \text{ mPa} \rightarrow 76 \text{ dB SPL}.$$

So, the rise to 78 dB happens within one time constant, but the return to 57 dB takes much longer, although there is only one time constant at work.

Nevertheless, many people will insist that they see two time constants from the measurement graph: an *attack time* of 5 ms and a *release time* of 30 ms. It will even get worse; the third example ahead will actually use two time constants. Then it will be possible to attribute two different values to the commonly used notion of a *release time*, depending on the perspective: looking at the measurement graph or at the decay of the observation window. To avoid confusion it is best to completely refrain from using the terms *attack time* and *release time*, and instead simply use the term *time constant* as defined with the observation window in an above subsection.

In summary, what has this first example shown so far? The level measurement using a short 5-ms time constant works well for the sinusoidal test signal. The result might encourage the choice of using even shorter time constants, thereby further reducing the settling time. However, for more complex test signals even a 5-ms time constant produces a disturbing measurement error. This is what we will look at next.

Measurement Error with Short Time Constants

Measurement errors become evident, as the test signal gets more complex. But why is another test signal needed at all? Many real signals from the acoustic environment are very different from a sinusoid. Voiced phonemes for instance exhibit regular pulses, as we have seen in Chapter 1 when looking at a speech signal. A pulsed signal, such as the one depicted in **Fig. 6–3a,** is a good test.

The pulsed signal consists of multiple cosine signals with frequencies of 100 Hz and integer multiples thereof. As a result, the pulses are 10 ms apart, as for voiced phonemes with a fundamental frequency of 100 Hz. Furthermore the sound pressure level of the new test signal also jumps between 55 and 80 dB SPL.

Figure 6–3b again shows the sound pressure level of the test signal along with the measured value—again using a 5 ms time constant. The diagram reveals a periodic measurement error, due to the test signal pulses that impact on the measured values. Let us imagine that the pulsed signal in **Fig. 6–3a** represents consecutive phonemes at 55 and 80 dB SPL; then the measured values should remain constant for the duration of each phoneme. They constantly change, however. In a WDRC system, this constantly changing level value propagates to the *compression characteristic* block that, in turn, produces a constantly changing gain value. The amplifier will consequently vary its gain within each phoneme, thus spoiling the sound quality.

The measurement value in **Fig. 6–3b** is designated as a *raw value* to indicate that the method needs some refinements to generate useful

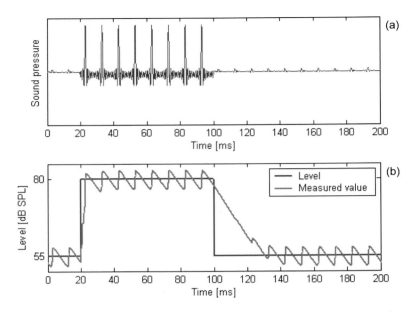

Figure 6–3   Level measurement using a short time
constant: **(a)** waveform of a
pulsed test signal and **(b)** sound
pressure level and
measurement value.

measurement values. The periodic measurement error actually is a real problem; it also occurs when measuring the sound pressure level of realistic signals.

Measurement Error with Asymmetric Time Constants

How is it possible to avoid the periodic measurement errors? The common practice is to use two different time constants:

◆ A short time constant when the sound pressure level increases

◆ A long time constant when the sound pressure level goes down

Example: While the sound pressure level increases, the 5-ms observation window from **Fig. 6–1a** is applied, but as soon as it sinks, the 100-ms observation window from **Fig. 6–1b** takes effect.

Using the time constants 5 ms and 100 ms as in the example yields the measurement values shown in **Fig. 6–4**:

◆ For the sinusoidal test signal in **Fig. 6–4a**

◆ For the pulsed test signal in **Fig. 6–4b**

Compared with the previous diagrams, the time axis now comprises a 10 times longer interval, that is, 2 s due to the longer 100-ms time constant for the falling sound pressure levels.

Using asymmetric time constants is effective: the periodic errors are gone, but there is a new measurement error. The measured value exceeds the sound pressure level by 2 dB for the sinusoidal test signal and by 8 dB for the pulsed signal. The size of this error depends on the specific signal waveform, so a fixed correction will only correct the error on average.

What causes this new error? It is difficult to explain the effect at this point, but we will see how it comes about in Chapter 13, where we will consider the calculation used in digital level measurement.

The measurement value depicted in **Fig. 6–4** is designated as a *peak value* because it is attached to a signal's maximum sound pressure level; interestingly enough, it actually exceeds it. The *peak value* also has the same behavior when measuring the sound pressure level of speech signals.

Measuring an Accurate Instantaneous Sound Pressure Level

The instantaneous measurement builds on the *raw value* as described in the second example. The refinement lies in applying a subsequent *nonlinear smoothing filter*. This filter suppresses small fluctuations in the measurement values,

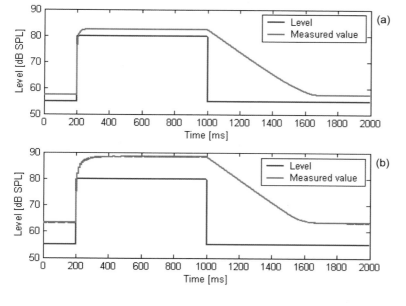

Figure 6–4   Level measurement using asymmetrical time constants, sound pressure level and measurement value: **(a)** for a sinusoidal test signal and **(b)** for a pulsed test signal.

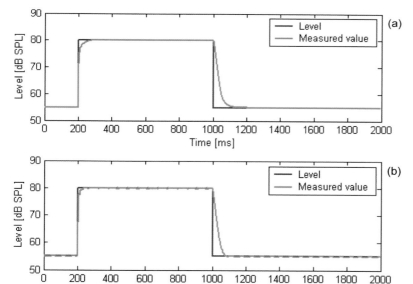

Figure 6–5   Level measurement using the instantaneous value method, sound pressure level and measurement value: **(a)** for a sinusoidal test signal and **(b)** for a pulsed test signal.

but follows large level changes without delay. In Chapter 13 I will present the calculations in detail; here we will just look at the results.

Figure 6–5 shows the measured values for the two test signals:

◆ The sinusoidal test signal in **Fig. 6–5a**
◆ The pulsed test signal in **Fig. 6–5b**

The measured value mostly matches the sound pressure level, apart from the periods that immediately follow a jump in level; the measurement then takes a short while to settle to the new value. Due to the immediate reaction, the measurement value in **Fig. 6–5** will be referred to as an *instantaneous value* from now on.

Level Measurement of Speech Signals

In this subsection, we will look at the measurement values that the different methods produce when applied to speech signals

1. For a single phoneme
2. For a complete word

The first example shows that the periodic measurement error also occurs with speech signals; the second example emphasizes the difference between the measurement of a *peak value* and an *instantaneous value*.

Measurement Values for a Single Phoneme

Figure 6–6a shows the sound pressure of a vowel over a 50-ms signal segment. Signal peaks appear at 14-ms intervals, corresponding to an extremely low-pitched male voice with a fundamental speech frequency of around 70 Hz. The low frequency causes the periodic measurement error to show up particularly well, even though the peaks in the waveform are only moderate.

Figure 6–6b shows three different level values measured by different methods:

♦ The *raw value*: measured with a short time constant of 5 ms

♦ The *segmental value*: measured with overlapping 10-ms segments

♦ The *instantaneous value*: measured with a short time constant and a subsequent smoothing filter

The *raw value* and the *segmental value* both exhibit the undesired periodic measurement error that **Fig. 6–3b** first showed for the pulse-shaped test signal. Using either of them in a WDRC system has the risk of spoiling the sound quality. By contrast, the *instantaneous value* runs smoothly – thanks to the smoothing filter.

Measurement Values for an Entire Word

Dealing with continuous speech, we will look at the measurement procedures that avoid the periodic measurement error, namely, we look at the *peak value* and the *instantaneous value*. Although the *segmental value* suffers from periodic errors, it still serves the purpose of a reference as it perfectly tracks the short-term sound pressure level of consecutive phonemes.

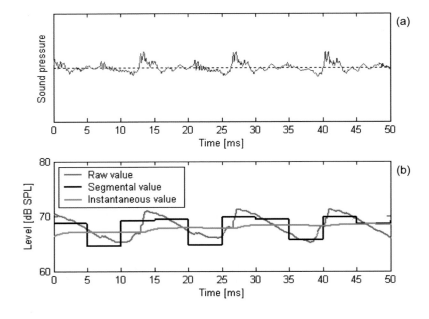

(a)

(b)

Figure 6–6   Level measurement of a single phoneme: **(a)** waveform of a single phoneme and **(b)** measurement values obtained with different methods.

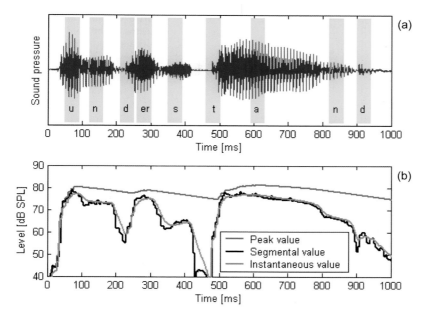

Figure 6–7 **Figure 6–7**   Level measurement for an entire word: **(a)** waveform of the word and **(b)** measurement values obtained with different methods.

Figure 6–7a shows the word "understand" that was first noted as one of the everyday signals in Chapter 1. **Figure 6–7b** shows the three different level values.

The *peak value* remains too high for the whole word and only changes by around 5 dB. This is due to using asymmetric time constants. A WDRC system using this method provides amplification that remains almost constant while someone speaks. In contrast, the *instantaneous value* follows the short-time sound pressure level of consecutive phonemes almost as well as the *segmental value*, which is perfect in this respect. The *instantaneous value* is thus ideal for very fast-acting WDRC. The hearing aid then amplifies the consonants by more and the vowels by less; thus higher consonant recognition is favored.

Using the *instantaneous value* might raise concerns about sound quality. In a later subsection, we will indeed see that it is not suitable for all WDRC schemes. The *instantaneous level value* has proven to be successful, however, as part of the WDRC scheme using the controllable lattice filter (Schaub & Leber, 2002) that we looked at in Chapter 5. Dillon et al (2003) found in a study that hearing impaired listeners gave this system the highest average scores for the sound quality of male and female voices as well as for piano music.

◆ Undesired Side Effects

Unfavorable temporal behavior adversely affects the sound quality of a WDRC system. We will consider the following two effects:

1. *Loss of spectral contrast*: occurs with fast-acting, multichannel WDRC
2. *Signal overshoot*: occurs when the gain decreases slowly after a sudden level increase

Loss of spectral contrast is also referred to as a form of *spectral smearing* that adversely affects speech recognition (Boothroyd et al, 1996).

Loss of Spectral Contrast

In this subsection, we will look again at the topic raised in Chapter 4: multichannel versus multiband WDRC. This time, however, let us assume that the processing schemes provide virtually perfect gain shaping capability as provided, for example, by the controllable finite impulse response (FIR) filter that we discussed in Chapter 5.

The test signal in this subsection is the word "shoe." The two phonemes in this word have totally different short-term spectra. **Figure 6–8a**

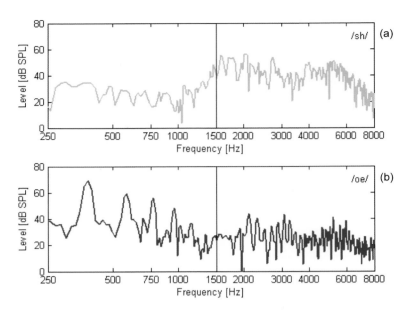

Figure 6–8   Spectra of the phonemes in the word "shoe": **(a)** sibilant /sh/ and **(b)** vowel /oe/.

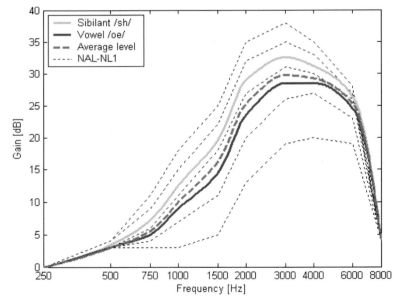

Figure 6–9   Gain curves of the two-band wide dynamic range compression system.

shows the spectrum of the sibilant /sh/ and **Fig. 6–8b** the spectrum of the vowel /oe/. The two phonemes differ in sound pressure level by around 10 dB and the spectrum of the sibilant rises with increasing frequency whereas the vowel's spectrum falls.

Multiband Wide Dynamic Range Compression

How does multiband WDRC amplify the signal? **Figure 6–9** shows the result for the previously used NAL-NL1 amplifications targets:

Table 6–1 Instantaneous Sound Pressure Levels

	Broadband	In Two Channels	
	0 – 8 kHz	0 – 1.5 kHz	1.5 – 8 kHz
Sibilant /sh/	65 dB SPL	58 dB SPL	64 dB SPL
Vowel /oe/	75 dB SPL	75 dB SPL	52 dB SPL

◆ For the sibilant /sh/ the gain curve lies between the targets for 60 and 70 dB SPL, in accordance with the instantaneous broadband sound pressure level of 65 dB SPL

◆ For the vowel sound /oe/ it lies between the targets for 70 and 80 dB SPL, in accordance with the level measurement of 75 dB SPL

Multiband WDRC also works when using an average sound-pressure level measured over the course of a few words. The amount of gain that the hearing aid generates then also depends on the previous words. In our example, the dashed red gain curve shows this case; the gain lies slightly below the 70 dB SPL targets for both phonemes of the word "shoe" and, in fact, does so for multiple consecutive words.

Multichannel Wide Dynamic Range Compression

The more channels a hearing aid has, and the faster it compresses the signal, the more it reduces the spectral contrast of the signal. The analysis here, however, covers only two channels; using the simplest example makes the cause of this effect stand out clearly.

Assume that the split frequency between the two channels is 1,500 Hz, as the vertical lines in **Figs. 6–8a** and **6–8b** show. As a result, almost the entire signal energy for the sibilant lies within the high-frequency channel, and the instantaneous value of the upper band signal reaches 64 dB SPL, as indicated in **Table 6–1**. The same goes for the vowel, but with respect to the low-frequency channel; almost the entire signal energy is in the lower band signal, and its instantaneous level value comes to 75 dB SPL. **Table 6–1** contains two further level measurements: 58 dB SPL in the low-frequency channel for the sibilant, and 52 dB SPL in the high-frequency channel for the vowel.

What effect do these level measurements have on a two-channel WDRC system? **Figure 6–10** shows the gain curves. The two-channel WDRC system amplifies the sibilant in the high-frequency channel by virtually the same amount

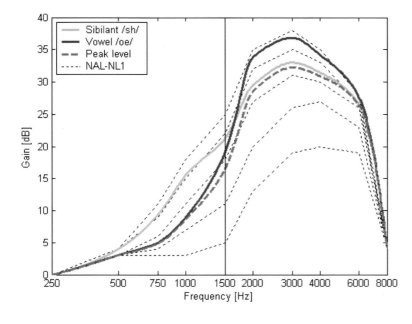

Figure 6–10 Gain curves of the two-channel wide dynamic range compression system.

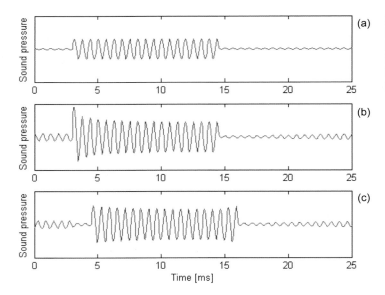

Figure 6–11   Signal overshoot:
(a) waveform of the input signal,
(b) output signal without compensating for the processing delay, and
(c) output signal with compensated processing delay.

as the multiband WDRC system. In the low-frequency channel, however, it applies more gain due to the lower level value in the low-frequency channel.

The behavior is reversed for the vowel sound. Here the two-channel WDRC system amplifies the low frequencies by the same amount as multiband WDRC, but the high frequencies receive more than 10 dB more gain; this is due to the more than 20 dB lower level value.

This simple example shows that two-channel WDRC amplifies both phonemes in a way that does not fit any targets. It consistently provides too much gain in one of the two frequency channels—always in the one containing less signal energy. This effect systematically smoothes out the spectral contrast, making it harder to tell different phonemes apart.

Fast WDRC in many channels makes the distortion audible and disturbing. There are two possible workarounds: *channel coupling* or slower control variables or both.

Channel coupling denotes the procedure of linking together multiple signal levels from narrow band signals, resulting in fewer signal levels that are valid for broader frequency ranges. In whatever way *channel coupling* is implemented, it always reduces the number of independent compression channels.

The other approach demands slower level measurements, such as the *peak value* taken from the level measurement using asymmet-

ric time constants. The dashed red curve in **Fig. 6–10** shows how much gain the two-channel WDRC system provides in this case. It is also different in relation to the targets—providing slightly too little gain in the low-frequency channel, and slightly too much again in the high-frequency channel. This is in accordance with the peak values of 76 and 67 dB SPL. In this case, however, only a small difference remains to multiband WDRC using a slowly varying broadband sound pressure level.

Signal Overshoot

The longer the observation window is, the more influence earlier sample values have on the level measurement of a digital signal, and the more the measurement value is delayed relative to the signal.

WDRC systems apply the measured sound pressure level to a compression characteristic and thereby define how much gain should be applied. If the sound pressure level increases suddenly, the output signal will overshoot; this is due to the time delay between the signal and its level measurement. After the jump in sound pressure level, it takes a certain time before the measured value reaches the new level. The hearing aid applies too much gain during this time period, initially as much gain as was correct for the lower sound pressure level before the jump, and then the gain gradually reduces.

Figure 6–11 illustrates the process for the ideal case of a short observation window. In particular,

- **Figure 6–11a** shows a short segment of a sinusoidal test signal.

- **Figure 6–11b** displays the amplified output signal. The output signal clearly overshoots at the start, although the gain adjusts to the new sound pressure level within 10 ms. Longer observation windows cause this undesirable effect to last even longer.

- **Figure 6–11c** depicts the output signal with diminished signal overshoot, as accomplished by delaying the acoustic signal relative to the gain that is applied to it. In this example, the additional delay is 1.5 ms.

Without synchronizing the signals, fast-acting WDRC runs the risk of producing signal overshoots at the beginning of each vowel, thus degrading sound quality. In Chapter 5, we noted that the two WDRC systems with controllable filters both provide for a *synchronization* block to implement the additional delay as a measure to preserve sound quality.

However, signal overshoot is less critical with a level measurement that uses asymmetric time constants. The resulting *peak level* avoids signal overshoots by keeping the measurement value constantly at maximum, but this slows the WDRC system down to virtually linear amplification.

◆ **Summary**

In this chapter, we first looked at the effect that the observation window has on the signal level measurement, and at the implications of using different time constants. We then considered different measurement methods and the errors

associated with them. We derived the level measurement with asymmetric time constants and the measurement of an instantaneous level value that enables the fastest-acting WDRC with highest sound quality.

Two undesired side effects were finally presented—side effects that are a consequence of unfavorable temporal behavior in WDRC systems: (1) fast compression in many frequency channels leads to loss of spectral contrast, and (2) signal overshoot occurs when the gain has a delay relative to the signal that is amplified.

References

Boothroyd A., Mulhearn B., Gong J., and Ostroff J. (1996). Effects of spectral smearing on phoneme and word recognition. Journal of the Acoustical Society of America, 100(3), 1807–1818.

Dillon H. (2001). Hearing aids, Thieme.

Dillon H., Keidser G., O'Brien A., and Silberstein H. (2003). Sound quality comparisons of advanced hearing aids. The Hearing Journal, 56(4), 30–40.

Edwards B. (2001). Application of Psychoacoustics to Audio Signal Processing. Proceedings of the 35th Asilomar Conference on Signals, Systems and Computers, November 5–7, Pacific Grove.

IEC 60118-2 (1983). Hearing aids. Part 2: Hearing aids with automatic gain control circuits, International Electrotechnical Commission, Geneva, Switzerland.

IEC 61672-1 (2002). Electroacoustics—sound level meters, Part 1: Specifications, International Electrotechnical Commission, Geneva, Switzerland.

Jenstad L.M., Seewald R.C., Cornelisse L.E., and Shantz J. (1999). Comparison of linear gain and wide dynamic range compression hearing aid circuits: aided speech perception measures. Ear & Hearing, 20(2), 117–126.

Kennedy E., Levitt H., Neuman A.C., and Weiss M. (1998). Consonant-vowel intensity ratios for maximizing consonant recognition by hearing-impaired listeners. Journal of the Acoustical Society of America, 103(2), 1098–1114.

Marriage, J. E., and Moore, B. C. (2003). New speech tests reveal benefit of wide-dynamic-range, fast-acting compression for consonant discrimination in children with moderate-to-profound hearing loss. International Journal of Audiology, 42(7), 418–425.

Mueller, H. G. (2000). What's the digital difference when it comes to patient benefit? The Hearing Journal, 53(3), 23–32.

Schaub, A., and Leber, R. (2002). Loudness-controlled processing of acoustic signals. United States Patent, US 6,370,255 B1, Apr. 9.

Smith, L. Z., and Levitt, H. (2000). Improving speech recognition in children: New hopes with digital hearing aids. The Hearing Journal, 53(3), 72–74.

Venema, T. (2006). Compression for clinicians (2nd ed.). Clifton Park, NY: Thomson Delmar Learning.

7

Acoustic Directionality

In this chapter, the capability of digital hearing instruments to adaptively suppress noise originating from behind or to the side of an individual is reviewed. The sections cover

1. *Static directionality*: as provided by a directional microphone having a front and a rear port or replicated by two omnidirectional microphones with electronic circuitry
2. *Adaptive directionality*: combines two omnidirectional microphones to form a directional pattern and adjusts the null direction toward the dominant signal source from the rear hemisphere
3. *Microphone matching*: reveals the adverse effect of microphones that differ in sensitivity and shows how to keep microphones matched during use

We will consider the ideal case of a directional microphone in the free field. Sound diffraction around the head, and reverberation in the surroundings reduce the benefit in normal listening conditions. As pointed out in Chapter 3, the *critical distance* is a useful concept to capture the impact of reverberation.

Nevertheless, many studies confirm the benefit of directional microphones (Ricketts & Hornsby, 2006; Bentler, 2005; Ricketts et al, 2001, 2003, 2005; Ricketts & Henry, 2002; Kochkin, 2000; Preves et al, 1999; Gravel et al, 1999; Ricketts & Dhar, 1999), even the limited benefit in case of reverberation (Ricketts & Hornsby, 2003). For an introduction to directional microphones, also see Csermak (2000).

◆ Static Directionality

Let us begin with two microphones that have equal sensitivity in all directions. **Figure 7–1** shows a suitable design for combining them to form a *static* directional microphone.

The diagram shows an example with a sound source to the rear of the two microphones. In this design, the rear microphone signal is delayed by a fixed time, T, and then subtracted from the front microphone signal. This gives a difference signal with a directional pattern dependent on the value chosen for T and also on the distance between the two microphones, and the frequency of the signal components. We will see shortly how these quantities interrelate. First, we will discuss the *cardioid* directional pattern that was mentioned in the overview of acoustic directionality in Chapter 3. Then we will consider how to generate other directional patterns.

Cardioid Directionality

A *cardioid pattern* cancels sound approaching from behind, namely, with an approach angle of 180 degrees. We will now look at the following three questions:

1. What value of T is needed to delay the rear microphone signal, such that sound from behind is cancelled?
2. What happens to sound from the front, with an approach angle of 0 degrees, under these conditions?

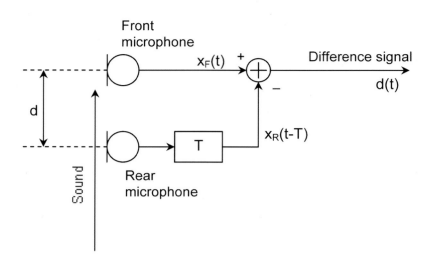

Figure 7–1 Construction of a directional microphone from two omnidirectional microphones.

3. What happens to sounds coming directly from the side, with an approach angle of +90 degrees or −90 degrees?

Sound from Behind

Sound arriving from behind reaches the rear microphone first, and takes an additional amount of time to reach the front microphone. Let us take the separation d between the two microphones to be 8.5 mm. In this case the sound, traveling at 340 m/s, takes an additional 25 μs to reach the front microphone. If the signal from the rear microphone is electronically delayed by 25 μs, then two identical signals are subtracted from one another. Theoretically, the difference signal is therefore zero, and the rear signal is completely cancelled. In practice, however, processing elements always slightly differ from one another and the rear signal is therefore just suppressed to a great extent. In a following section, we will actually consider the impact of microphones that have different sensitivity.

Sound from the Front

We now look at what happens to signals from the front, using the electronic delay of 25 μs. As an example, we will consider a previously used test signal: a signal that is made up of four sinusoidal signals, each of 75 dB SPL amplitude, which was introduced in Chapter 1. The frequencies of the sinusoids are 500 Hz, 1 kHz, 2 kHz, and 4 kHz; they are one octave apart from one another.

Figure 7–2a shows two signals:

◆ The signal from the front microphone $x_F(t)$

◆ The 25 μs delayed signal from the rear microphone $x_R(t-T)$

The short 2-ms segment shows that signal $x_F(t)$ leads signal $x_R(t-T)$ by a total of 50 μs: 25 μs is needed for the signal to get from the front to the rear microphone, and the additional 25 μs is the electronic delay subsequently applied to the rear microphone signal.

Figure 7–2b shows the difference signal d(t). Comparing it to the two microphone signals in **Fig. 7–2a**, we see that the waveform has slightly changed. This is so because signals approaching from the front do not pass unchanged through a directional microphone. The directional microphone has the effect of a high-pass filter, as the signal spectra in **Fig. 7–3** show

◆ For an approach angle of 0 degrees in **Fig. 7–3a**

◆ For an approach angle of ±90 degrees in **Fig. 7–3b**

Initially, all of the tones have amplitudes of 75 dB SPL. After passing through the directional microphone the level of each tone is 6 dB less than the level of the tone with a frequency one octave higher. This high-pass filter effect causes the waveform to change and reduces the sound pressure level as well. With additional circuitry

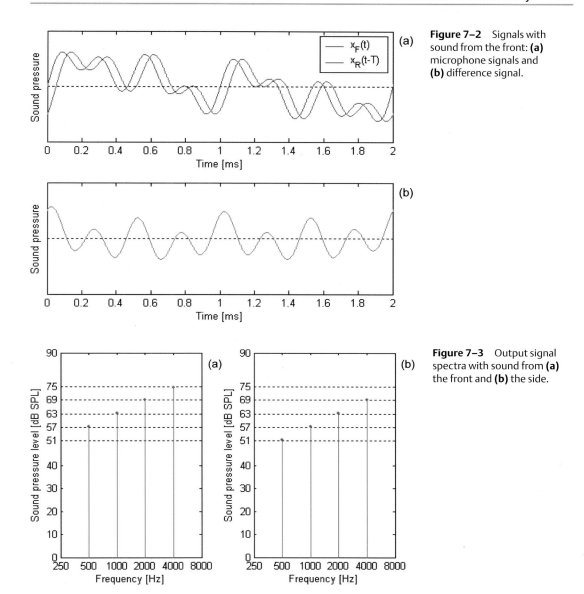

Figure 7–2 Signals with sound from the front: **(a)** microphone signals and **(b)** difference signal.

Figure 7–3 Output signal spectra with sound from **(a)** the front and **(b)** the side.

it is possible, however, to compensate for this effect – at least partially.

Sound from the Side

Next we look at signals approaching exactly from the side, that is, at an approach angle of ± 90 degrees. In this case the sound reaches both microphones simultaneously. As shown in **Fig.**

7–4a, signal $x_F(t)$ now only leads signal $x_R(t-T)$ by 25 μs, the electronic delay of the rear microphone signal. The difference signal $d(t)$ in **Fig. 7–4b** resembles that from **Fig. 7–2b**; this time, however, the sound pressure variation is smaller.

The spectrum in **Fig. 7–3b** shows that all of the tones produce a 6 dB lower level than in the case of the test signal approaching from the front, and that the directional microphone also

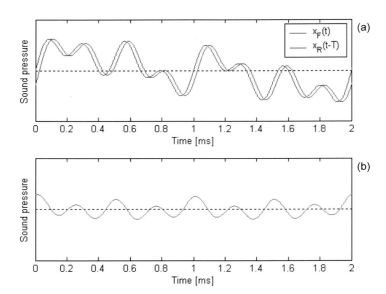

Figure 7–4   Signals with sound from the side: **(a)** microphone signals and **(b)** difference signal.

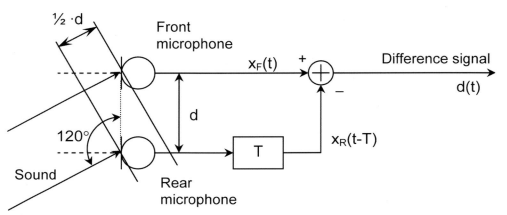

Figure 7–5   Sound approaching at 120 degrees.

acts as a high-pass filter for signals approaching from the side.

Let us summarize the sensitivity in the three directions analyzed so far.

◆ Sound from the front: 0 dB reference
◆ Sound from the side: −6 dB with respect to sound from the front
◆ Sound from the rear: completely suppressed

These three cases correspond to the *cardioid pattern* that was discussed in Chapter 3. I will refrain from examining additional approach angles, and look instead at how to generate different directional patterns.

Other Directional Patterns

How is it possible to generate other directional patterns – supercardioid or hypercardioid, for example, as discussed in Chapter 3? There are two main approaches: one obvious and one which, although more unusual, is especially suited to producing *adaptive* directionality.

The obvious solution is to delay the rear microphone signal by a smaller amount, for example by $T = 12.5$ μs. As **Fig. 7–5** shows, this configuration will completely suppress signals approaching at an angle of 120 degrees. The sound coming from this angle only needs to cover an extra distance of $^1/_2 \cdot d = 4.25$ mm to

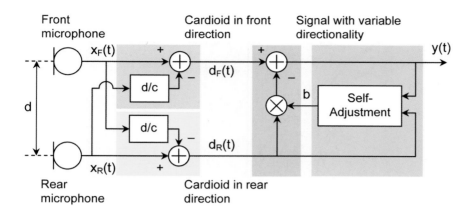

Figure 7-6 Block diagram of adaptive directionality.

reach the front microphone. This also takes 12.5 μs, generating two identical signals that are again subtracted from one another.

With no electronic delay, the directional microphone suppresses sound that reaches both microphones simultaneously, namely, sound with approach angles of ±90 degrees.

Therefore, we can conclude that choosing a value of T between 0 and 25 μs suppresses signals with approach angles between ±90 degrees and 180 degrees.

In the next section, I will present the alternative method for producing different directional patterns, and show how to use it for *adaptive* directionality.

◆ Adaptive Directionality

Most hearing instruments use a state-of-the-art procedure (Elko, 1995) to implement *adaptive* directionality. The analysis here divides into the following:

1. *Block diagram*: provides an overview of how the circuitry processes the front and rear microphone signals to achieve adaptive directionality

2. *Programmable directionality*: illustrates how to set the null direction, that is, the approach angle at which the directional microphone completely suppresses sound

3. *Self-adjustment*: reveals the strategy that allows the directional microphone to adjust permanently the null direction itself

Block Diagram

The block diagram in **Fig. 7-6** is split into four parts marked by different colors. Each part produces a distinct output signal, as follows:

1. The *green* part produces the difference signal $d_F(t)$, featuring a *front-cardioid* pattern.

2. The *yellow* part generates the difference signal $d_R(t)$, featuring a *rear-cardioid* pattern.

3. The *blue* part produces the output signal $y(t)$, featuring a *variable directional pattern*.

4. The *red* part calculates the factor, b, which defines the null direction.

The factor b deals with setting the null direction and is addressed in a following subsection.

Front-Cardioid Pattern

The difference signal $d_F(t)$ is generated by the delay-and-subtract method used for *static* directionality as discussed in an above section. To produce the *cardioid pattern*, the delay is set to d/c, where d is the distance between the front and rear microphone and c is the speed of sound, 340 m/s.

Rear-Cardioid Pattern

Reversing the roles of the two microphones produces the difference signal $d_R(t)$. The front microphone signal is delayed and then subtracted from the rear microphone signal. The delay is again set to d/c, resulting in a *cardioid* pattern directed toward the rear.

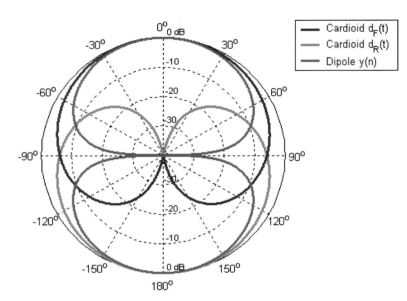

—	Cardioid $d_F(t)$
—	Cardioid $d_R(t)$
—	Dipole $y(n)$

Figure 7–7   Bipolar directional pattern.

Variable Directional Pattern

The output signal y(t) is generated as a combination of the *front-cardioid* signal $d_F(t)$ and *rear-cardioid* signal $d_R(t)$. The processing scheme first multiplies the *rear-cardioid* signal $d_R(t)$ by the factor *b*, and then subtracts the result from the *front-cardioid* signal $d_F(t)$:

$$y(t) = d_F(t) - b \cdot d_R(t) \qquad \text{(Eq. 7–1)}$$

The resulting directionality pattern depends on the value of factor *b*.

Programmable Directionality

If the self-adjustment block were missing in **Fig. 7–6**, then it would still be possible to generate different fixed directional patterns, by varying the value of factor *b*. We will look at directional patterns that different values for *b* generate

$b = 0$
$b = 1$
$b = 0.5$

Factor *b* = 0.   This is the simplest case. The *front-cardioid* signal $d_F(t)$ passes through unchanged to the output. The output signal y(t) therefore has the *cardioid* pattern.

Factor *b* = 1.   We will consider this case with the help of **Fig. 7–7.** The blue curve shows the *front-cardioid* pattern of the signal $d_F(t)$ and the green curve shows the *rear-cardioid* pattern of the signal $d_R(t)$.

The two directional patterns intersect at the approach angles of +90 degrees and −90 degrees. Consequently, signals coming from ±90 degrees have the same amplitude, and the directional microphone cancels them by subtracting one signal from the other. The red curve shows the resulting directional pattern that is also known as a *bipolar* response.

Factor *b* = 0.5.   **Figure 7–8** illustrates this case. The blue curve again shows the *front-cardioid* pattern of the signal $d_F(t)$, while the green curve shows the *rear-cardioid* pattern of the signal $d_R(t)$ multiplied by factor *b* = 0.5, that is, attenuated by 6 dB. This time the two directional patterns intersect at approach angles of +110 degrees and −110 degrees. Therefore, signals coming from ±110 degrees have the same amplitude, and again the directional microphone cancels them by subtracting one signal from the other. The red curve shows the resulting directional pattern that is also known as a *hypercardioid* response.

The three examples have shown that changing the value of factor *b* produces differing

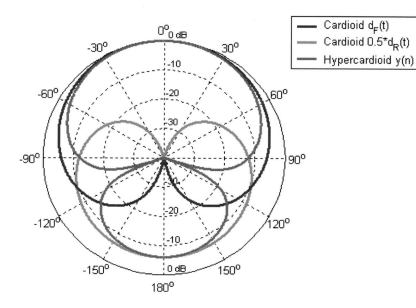

Figure 7–8 Hypercardioid directional pattern.

directional patterns. The values $b = 0$ and $b = 1$ suppress signals at approach angles of 180 degrees and ± 90 degrees, respectively. They present the minimum and maximum admissible values for factor b — and values in between cause the directional microphone to suppress sound coming from intermediate angles. What remains is to explain how the directional microphone can optimize factor b itself to cancel the unwanted noise.

Self-adjustment

An example is best suited to illustrate the idea of how the self-adjustment mechanism works: a speech signal approaches from the front with an approach angle of 0 degrees, and an additional noise source produces sound approaching from the rear, at an angle of 120 degrees. Now we will look in turn at

1. The microphone signals $x_F(t)$ and $x_R(t)$
2. The *front-cardioid* signal $d_F(t)$ and the *rear-cardioid* signal $d_R(t)$
3. The output signal $y(t)$
4. Finally, comparing the signals $d_R(t)$ and $y(t)$ will reveal how a directional microphone can set the value of factor b itself.

The Microphone Signals. Figure 7–9 shows the two microphone signals:

- The front microphone signal $x_F(t)$ in **Fig. 7–9a**
- The rear microphone signal $x_R(t)$ in **Fig. 7–9b**

The noise signal is so strong that it completely obscures the speech signal.

The Front and Rear Cardioid Signals. Figure 7–10 shows the two signals with a *cardioid* pattern:

- The *front-cardioid* signal $d_F(t)$ in **Fig. 7–10a**
- The *rear-cardioid* signal $d_R(t)$ in **Fig. 7–10b**

The *front-cardioid* signal $d_F(t)$ exhibits the word "understand" from Chapter 1. However, the noise signal is still strong enough to mask the stop consonants /t/ and /d/.

The *rear-cardioid* signal $d_R(t)$ contains only noise because its *rear-cardioid* pattern completely suppresses the speech signal coming from the front.

Comparing the *cardioid* signals with the microphone signals, we again see a reduction in the sound pressure level because the directional microphone acts as a high-pass filter. It is possible to largely compensate for this effect by applying a low-pass filter to the directional signals and a few dB of amplification. The diagrams ahead will show signals that include this compensation.

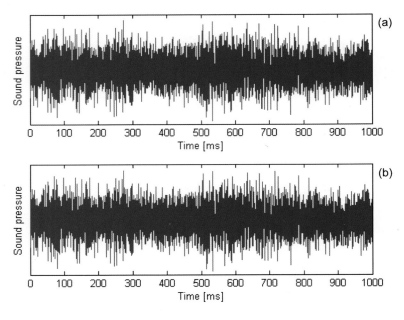

Figure 7–9   Microphone signals of speech in noise: **(a)** front microphone and **(b)** rear microphone.

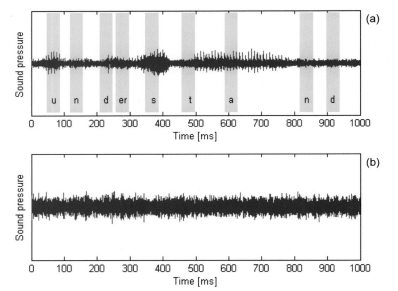

Figure 7–10   Difference signals of speech in noise, with cardioid patterns: **(a)** in front direction and **(b)** in rear direction.

The Output Signal. We will observe the output signal y(t) for the three different directional patterns shown in **Figure 7–11**. The factor b takes the value 0.13, 0.33, and 0.53, respectively. If $b = 0.13$, then the directional microphone cancels signals with an approach angle of ± 140 degrees, whereas if $b = 0.53$, then sound from ± 108 degrees will be cancelled. In both cases, the directional microphone attenuates the unwanted noise by around 16 dB; the remaining noise, however, still covers the stop consonants, as **Fig. 7–12** shows

- For $b = 0.13$ in **Fig. 7–12a**
- For $b = 0.53$ in **Fig. 7–12b**

Only choosing $b = 0.33$ causes the directional microphone to completely suppress all the

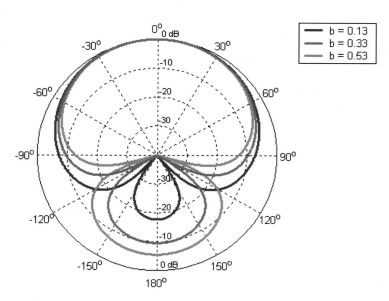

Figure 7–11 Different directional patterns for varying values of the factor *b*.

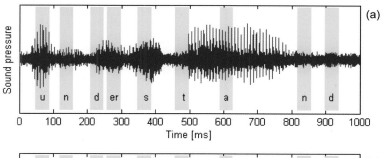

(a)

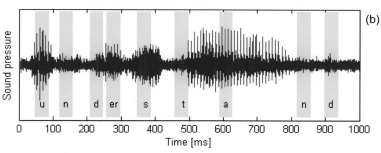

(b)

Figure 7–12 Output signals with nonoptimized values of *b*: **(a)** *b* = 0.13 and **(b)** *b* = 0.53.

noise approaching at an angle of 120 degrees. **Figure 7–13a** shows the output signal y(t) in this case, and now again exhibits the waveform of the stop consonants /t/ and /d/.

The Control Signals. **Figure 7–13b** shows the *rear-cardioid* signal $d_R(t)$ and the output signal y(t) for a 5-ms time segment, from 815 ms to 820 ms. As previously mentioned, the *rear-cardioid* signal $d_R(t)$ consists entirely of

unwanted noise. An optimized value for factor *b* causes the correct amount of noise to be subtracted from the *front-cardioid* signal $d_F(t)$, thus producing an output signal y(t) with the unwanted noise completely removed. In this case y(t) only shows the waveform of the nasal /n/.

Figure 7–14 again shows the signals $d_R(t)$ and y(t), but this time for the nonoptimized values of factor *b*.

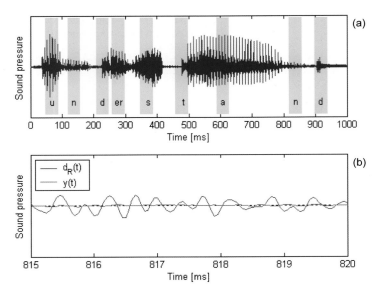

Figure 7–13   Signals with optimized factor b: **(a)** output signal and **(b)** control signals.

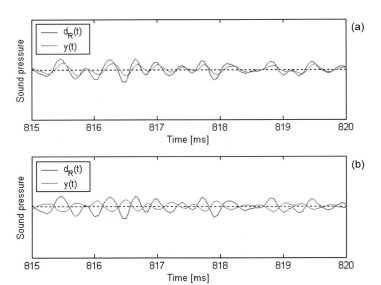

Figure 7–14   Control signals with nonoptimized values of b: **(a)** $b = 0.13$ and **(b)** $b = 0.53$.

◆ For $b = 0.13$ in **Fig. 7–14a**
◆ For $b = 0.53$ in **Fig. 7–14b**

With $b = 0.13$ the directional microphone subtracts too little, so the output signal $y(t)$ still contains a component of the unwanted noise. With $b = 0.53$, however, the directional microphone subtracts too much. As a result, the unwanted noise still appears in the output signal, but with an inverse sign, namely, with opposite phase.

This suggests a way in which the directional microphone can automatically adjust factor b to find the optimum value, a *sign rule*.

If the *rear-cardioid* signal $d_R(t)$ and the output signal $y(t)$ have the same sign, then increase factor b by a small amount; if they have different signs, then reduce factor b by a similarly small amount.

Using this *sign rule*, the value of b will gradually approach its ideal value. Once the optimum

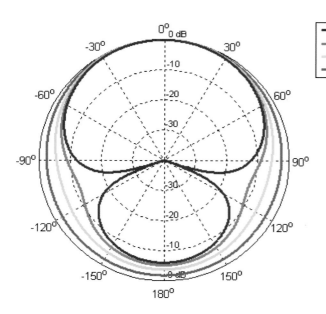

— 0 dB	
— 0.5 dB	
— 1 dB	
— 2 dB	

Figure 7–15 Directional patterns for microphones with different sensitivities.

value is reached, the signs will tend to agree and disagree equally often, and b will remain nearly constant.

In practice, a self-adjustment block updates factor b in each sampling period. To this end it calculates small adjustment values as a function of the values of signals $d_R(t)$ and $y(t)$, compliant with the *sign rule*. The quantitative aspect of the calculation is beyond the scope of this book. It is interesting to note, however, that this adaptive process has proved itself in practice, even when the signals have less ideal properties than in this example.

◆ **Microphone Matching**

The analysis, until now, implicitly assumed that the two microphones exhibit equal sensitivity. If they do not, then the directional pattern worsens significantly. **Figure 7–15** illustrates the *hypercardioid* pattern for perfectly matching microphones as well as for a mismatch of 0.5, 1, and 2 dB, respectively. The deviation is enormous.

In practice, directional hearing aids always use well-matched microphones. Sensitivity may change over time though. To ensure a reliable directional pattern thus requires continuous calibration.

Figure 7–16 shows how to keep microphones matched while the hearing instrument is operating. The front and rear microphone signals go to *level measurement* blocks and their output signals feed a *comparator*. The output signal of the *comparator* causes the subsequent *up/down counter* to count upwards or downwards, depending on which signal level is higher. Due to its limited number range, the *up/down counter* is eventually subject to an *overflow* or an *underflow*. In either event, a signal goes to the two subsequent *up/down counters* that each holds a factor to multiply with its respective microphone signal.

Let us see what happens in the following three cases:

1. The two microphones have *equal* sensitivity: Either microphone signal has higher and lower level half of the time. The *comparator* causes the first *up/down counter* to count upward and downward equally often, no *overflow* occurs and no *underflow*. The factors in the last two *up/down counters* remain constant.

2. The front microphone has *higher* sensitivity than the rear microphone: The front microphone signal mostly has a higher level, the *comparator* causes the *up/down counter* to mostly count upward, eventually an *overflow* occurs. This event slightly decreases

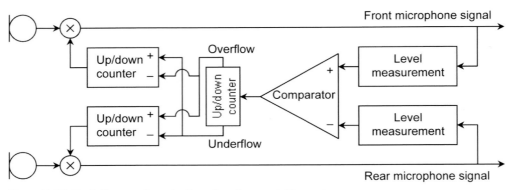

Figure 7–16 Block diagram of an adaptive microphone matching system.

the factor that multiplies with the front microphone signal and at the same time slightly increases the factor that multiplies with the rear microphone signal. This process repeats itself until the two factors effectively correct the microphone mismatch.

3. The front microphone has *lower* sensitivity than the rear microphone: The front microphone signal mostly has a lower level, the *comparator* causes the *up/down counter* to mostly count downward; eventually an *underflow* occurs. This event slightly increases the factor that multiplies with the front microphone signal and at the same time slightly decreases the factor that multiplies with the rear microphone signal. This process repeats itself until the two factors effectively correct the microphone mismatch.

This calibration mechanism is again an adaptive algorithm that effectively removes a slight microphone mismatch of a few dB. It is useless, however, in the case of a big sensitivity difference when one of the microphones is blocked, for example by hairspray, debris, etc.

In practice, it is possible to extend the mechanism to provide more than just one multiplier to each microphone signal. This extension results in an adaptive filter that may as well adaptively correct spectral tilt. This topic is beyond the scope of this book, however.

◆ Summary

In this chapter, we first looked at how to combine two equally sensitive microphones in such a way that they form a *static* directional microphone. Then the focus was on combining two such *static* microphones, with the aim of creating an *adaptive* directional microphone. The *adaptive* directional microphone has the potential of continuously canceling unwanted noise from the side or rear. To this end, a method was presented that adjusts the microphone's directional pattern accordingly.

Finally, we explored the effect that microphones with different sensitivities have on the directional pattern, and how it is possible to keep microphones permanently matched while the hearing instrument is operating.

References

Bentler, R. A. (2005). Effectiveness of directional microphones and noise reduction schemes in hearing aids: A systematic review of the evidence. Journal of the American Academy of Audiology, 16(7), 473–484.

Csermak, B. (2000). A primer on a dual microphone directional system. The Hearing Review, 7(1), 56–60.

Elko, G. W., and Nguyen Pong, A.-T. (1995). A simple adaptive first-order differential microphone. In Proceedings of the 1995 IEEE ASSP Workshop on Applications of Signal Processing to Audio and Acoustics (pp. 169–172). Piscataway, NJ: IEEE.

Gravel, J. S., Fausel, N., Liskow, C., and Chobot J. (1999). Children's speech recognition in noise using omnidirectional and dual-microphone hearing aid technology. Ear & Hearing, 20(1), 1–11.

Kochkin, S. (2000). Customer satisfaction with single and multiple microphone digital hearing aids. The Hearing Review, 7(11), 24–29.

Preves, D. A., Sammeth C. A., and Wynne, M. K. (1999). Field trial evaluations of a switched directional/omnidirectional in-the-ear hearing instrument. Journal of the American Academy of Audiology, 10(5), 273–284.

Ricketts, T., and Dhar, S. (1999). Comparison of performance across three directional hearing aids. Journal of the American Academy of Audiology, 10(4), 180–189.

Ricketts, T., and Henry, P. (2002). Evaluation of an adaptive, directional-microphone hearing aid. International Journal of Audiology, 41(2), 100–112.

Ricketts, T., Henry, P., and Gnewikow, D. (2003). Full time directional versus user selectable microphone modes in hearing aids. Ear & Hearing, 24(5), 424–439.

Ricketts, T. A., and Hornsby, B. W. (2003). Distance and reverberation effects on directional benefit. Ear & Hearing, 24(6), 472–484.

Ricketts, T. A., and Hornsby, B. (2006). Directional hearing aid benefit in listeners with severe hearing loss. International Journal of Audiology, 45(3), 190–197.

Ricketts, T. A., Hornsby, B. W. Y., and Johnson, E. E. (2005). Adaptive directional benefit in the near field: Competing sound angle and level effects. Seminars in Hearing, 26, 59–69.

Ricketts, T., Lindley, G., and Henry, P. (2001). Impact of compression and hearing aid style on directional hearing aid benefit and performance. Ear & Hearing, 22(4), 348–361.

8

Noise Reduction

In this chapter, we address how digital hearing aids suppress noise that maintains a more or less constant sound pressure level over time, such as noise in a car or train, for example. In contrast to the previous chapter, this noise reduction is independent of the approach angle that the noise comes from. The sections in this chapter cover

1. *Overview of adaptive noise reduction*: illustrates the effect on speech in noise and presents two variants for implementing a noise reduction system
2. *The various processing steps*: measuring band signal levels, determining modulation, defining attenuation, and attenuating the band signals
3. *Additional options*: speed of noise reduction, dependence on sound pressure level, and interaction with WDRC

Several studies have investigated the benefit of noise reduction systems. They confirm a significant improvement in listening comfort, but no impact on speech recognition scores (Mueller et al, 2006; Ricketts & Hornsby, 2005; Walden et al, 2000; Boymans & Dreschler, 2000) – with the exception of the reports by Bray and Nilsson (2001) and Bray and Wilson (2000), which also claim significant improvement to speech intelligibility. For further discussion on noise reduction, see also Bentler and Chiou (2006), Schum (2003), and Levitt (2001).

◆ Overview of Adaptive Noise Reduction

Today's digital hearing aids suppress noise by analyzing and processing the acoustic signal in many bands – up to 64. The analysis here, however, uses only three bands, as this is sufficient to illustrate how the principle works.

The block diagram in **Fig. 8–1** shows how the noise reduction system processes the acoustic signal. The diagram includes three filters, a low-pass, a band-pass, and a high-pass filter, to split the input signal x(t) into band signals. In each frequency band the processing scheme then determines the optimum attenuation for that band signal, and loads this value into a programmable amplifier. The three amplifiers attenuate the band signals accordingly, and finally the processing scheme recombines the attenuated signals to form the output signal y(t).

Figure 8–2a shows a typical example of speech in noise. Yellow bars in the range 0.5 to 1.5 second indicate the individual phonemes in the word "understand" that is familiar from the everyday acoustic signals presented in Chapter 1. The signal before and after the word "understand" consists entirely of noise.

Figure 8–2b illustrates the result of the simple three-band processing. The output signal y(t) has a lower sound pressure level that makes it sound softer. Also, the structure of the

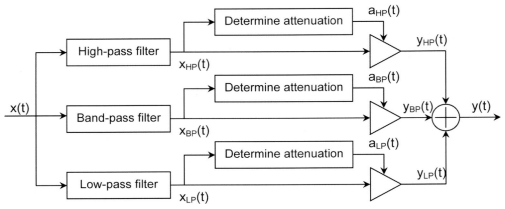

Figure 8–1   Block diagram of a noise reduction system using band signals.

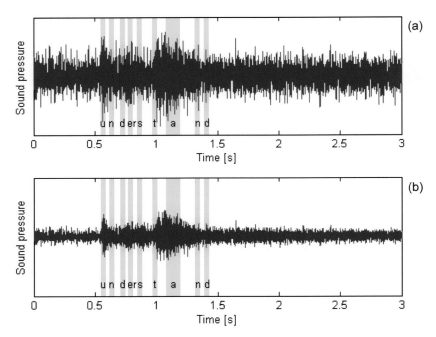

Figure 8–2   Effect of adaptive noise reduction: **(a)** input signal – speech in noise and **(b)** output signal – speech with suppressed noise.

word "understand" stands out more clearly than in the input signal.

Before concluding this section, we will take a quick look at another potential architecture. **Figure 8–3** shows how a controllable filter can be used to achieve the same processing. This approach again determines how much to attenuate in each frequency band, and then applies this attenuation using a controllable FIR filter. It processes the acoustic signal as a whole, without splitting it into band signals. This method has some benefits, especially in relation to

numerical precision and power consumption. In Chapter 12, I will present a practical implementation in detail (Schaub, 2003).

◆ The Various Processing Steps

The first operation in the block diagram of **Fig. 8–1** consists of splitting the input signal into band signals. **Figure 8–4** shows the three band signals from our example. As is common in reality, the

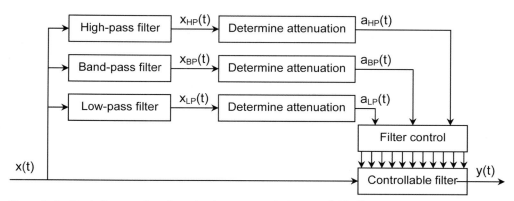

Figure 8–3   Block diagram of a noise reduction system using a controllable filter.

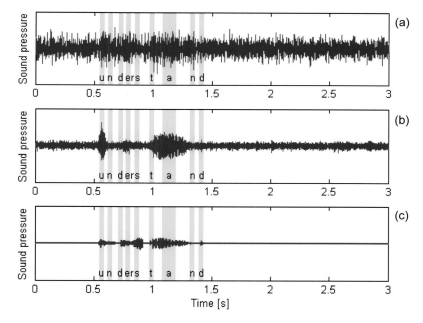

Figure 8–4   Speech and noise in band signals: **(a)** 0 Hz to 500 Hz, **(b)** 500 Hz to 2 kHz, and **(c)** 2 kHz to 8 kHz.

noise in our example masks the speech signal most in the frequency range below 500 Hz, significantly less in the mid-frequency range, and has a minimal effect above 2 kHz.

Next, we will look at how to find the optimum attenuation for each band signal. The block diagram in **Fig. 8–5** shows the three steps to take for each band signal.

1. Measure the level, p(t)
2. Determine how much this level varies over a short time segment, giving the modulation m(t)

3. Select the attenuation a(t) as a function of the modulation

One more processing step is finally needed: attenuate each band signal by the value of a(t) and add the attenuated signals to form the output signal y(t).

Measuring Band Signal Levels

We have already looked at how to measure signal levels in Chapter 6. An accurate instantaneous sound pressure level is also suitable for noise reduction.

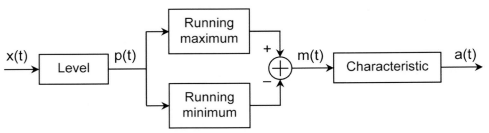

Figure 8–5   Block diagram of circuitry for defining attenuation.

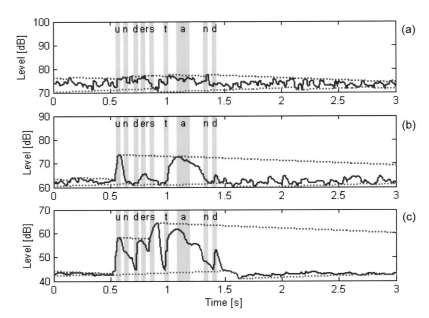

Figure 8–6   Signal level with running maxima and minima in all three frequency bands: **(a)** 0 Hz to 500 Hz, **(b)** 500 Hz to 2 kHz, and **(c)** 2 kHz to 8 kHz.

Determining Modulation

The block diagram in **Fig. 8–5** shows in detail how to find the modulation in two steps:

1. Calculate the short-term running maxima and minima of the signal level in each frequency band.
2. Take the differences between the running maxima and minima.

Figure 8–6 shows the signal levels in the three frequency ranges, as well as the running maxima and minima, represented in the diagrams by the green and red dotted curves.

How is it possible to determine the running maximum? The calculation is iterative, that is, repeats itself at each sampling period, selecting the *larger* of two values:

◆ Either the previous running maximum *minus* a tiny constant
◆ Or the current signal level

In this way, the running maximum decreases gradually while it exceeds the current signal level, but instantly responds to a new peak.

Acquiring the running minimum proceeds by analogy, taking the *smaller* of two values:

◆ Either the previous running minimum *plus* a tiny constant
◆ Or the current signal level

Here the running minimum increases gradually while it is below the current signal level, but instantly responds to a new low.

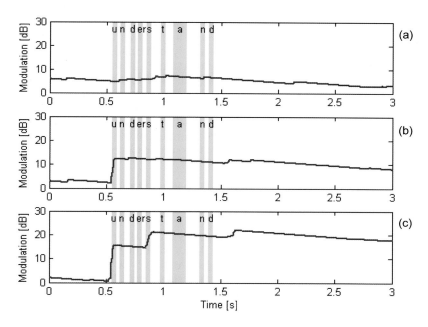

Figure 8–7   Modulation in all three frequency bands: **(a)** 0 Hz to 500 Hz, **(b)** 500 Hz to 2 kHz, and **(c)** 2 kHz to 8 kHz.

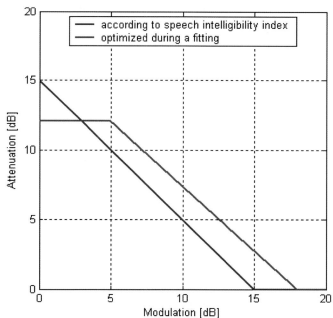

Figure 8–8   Transfer characteristics for optimum attenuation as a function of modulation.

Figure 8–7 shows the resulting modulations m(t) of the signals from each frequency band. Below 500 Hz the modulation varies only slightly when speech sets in. In the middle band, however, the modulation suddenly increases by 10 dB. In the high-frequency range, the modulation increases by 15 dB at the beginning and by a further 5 dB in the middle of the word "understand." After the word, apart from small random variations, the modulation again decreases in each frequency band, and will eventually reach the values seen prior to the start of the word.

Defining Attenuation

Once the modulation, m(t), is determined, the next step involves calculating the desired attenuation. **Figure 8–8** shows two possible functions:

1. The blue curve shows the 15-dB rule as derived from the speech intelligibility model (ANSI, 1997) in Chapter 3.
2. The green curve shows a typical transfer characteristic, obtained when optimizing the hearing aid in a field test.

According to the 15-dB rule, band signals with a modulation greater than 15 dB pass unchanged through the noise reduction scheme. Band signals with lower modulation will be attenuated by the difference between 15 dB and their own modulation.

Examples:

Modulation: 10 dB → Attenuation: 5 dB

Modulation: 5 dB → Attenuation: 10 dB

The green curve in **Fig. 8–8** allows all band signals with a modulation greater than 18 dB to pass unchanged. For modulation values less than 18 dB, the attenuation steadily increases, until it reaches the maximum attenuation of 12 dB, when modulation is 5 dB or less. To further optimize the hearing aid performance, such transfer characteristics can be set differently for the different frequency bands.

Figure 8–9 shows the attenuation according to the 15-dB rule. In the low-frequency band, the attenuation is only marginally reduced during the word "understand." In the mid-frequency band, however, the attenuation is significantly reduced. In the high-frequency band, the modulation increases by more than 20 dB, thereby allowing the signal to pass through unchanged – not just for the duration of the word, but also for an additional few seconds afterward.

Attenuating the Band Signals and Forming the Output Signal

Once the attenuation, a(t) is determined, the next step involves attenuating the band signals. **Figure 8–10** shows all of the processed band signals when applying the 15-dB rule to our example. Comparing these signals with the ones before attenuation in **Figure 8–4** makes it clear: the noise reduction procedure reduces the sound pressure the most in the low-frequency band where the noise causes the most disturbance.

◆ Additional Options

So far, we have looked at the basics of noise reduction, which, in practice, can be applied in

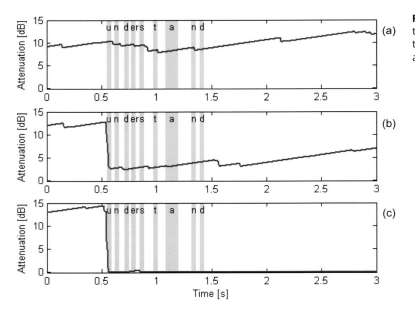

Figure 8–9 Attenuation in all three frequency bands: **(a)** 0 Hz to 500 Hz, **(b)** 500 Hz to 2 kHz, and **(c)** 2 kHz to 8 kHz.

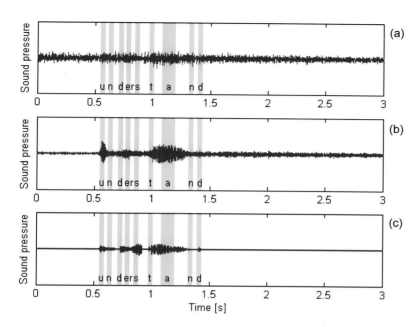

Figure 8–10 The attenuated band signals: **(a)** 0 Hz to 500 Hz, **(b)** 500 Hz to 2 kHz, and **(c)** 2 kHz to 8 kHz.

several different ways. In this final section, we will consider three questions.

1. How fast should the noise reduction system attenuate when the modulation decreases? And how fast should it remove the attenuation when the modulation increases?

2. Should the noise reduction system handle monotonic noise of different sound pressure levels in the same way?

3. How should noise reduction work in combination with wide dynamic range compression (WDRC)?

Speed of Noise Reduction

The noise reduction system in our example removes attenuation rapidly as modulation increases, at the onset of speech, for example. On the other hand, the attenuation increases only gradually as the modulation decreases – during a pause, for instance. But there are also other options to the temporal behavior.

In Chapter 6, we looked at the temporal behavior of WDRC. Two ways were given to measure sound pressure level for use in WDRC, as a peak value or as an instantaneous value. With noise reduction, it is also possible to measure an instantaneous modulation value

and to react quickly, both when modulation increases and decreases.

To determine an instantaneous modulation, it is no longer necessary to calculate the running maximum of the signal; it is instead possible to use the rapidly changing signal level directly. As with fast WDRC it is important that the signals – in this case attenuation and band signal – are well aligned in time to maintain good sound quality.

Dependence on Sound Pressure Level

The analysis, so far, attenuates soft and loud noise equally when they contain the same amount of modulation. This can prove a disadvantage in practice. Soft monotonic sounds could contain important information that the hearing aid wearer would then miss. It makes sense, therefore, to gradually attenuate signals less when their sound pressure level falls below a certain threshold.

Interaction with WDRC

Noise reduction and WDRC both affect the amount of amplification or attenuation that is applied to individual signal components. The overall effect depends on which is applied first.

The 15-dB rule presupposes that the unwanted noise is first suppressed, and then the cleaned signal is amplified according to the needs of the individual hearing aid wearer. If the compression ratio is 2:1 throughout, then it would be possible to swap the processing steps around and achieve the same noise reduction effect by applying only half the attenuation – in other words: with a 7.5-dB rule. However, the curvilinear compression characteristics used for WDRC in today's digital hearing aids favor the first approach: apply noise reduction first and WDRC afterward.

In practice, there is one further aspect to consider: if the two processing stages are really performed consecutively, then the total processing cost will increase as well as the processing delay. It is therefore advantageous to combine the two processes arithmetically, taking care to maintain the preferred sequence. It is again possible to achieve this combination either by splitting the signal into band signals or by using a controllable filter (Schaub, 2004).

◆ Summary

In this chapter, we familiarized ourselves with the concept of adaptively suppressing monotonic noise, using a simplified example. We first looked at a typical processing architecture that splits the input signal into band signals. Then, we considered a different implementation using a controllable filter. The analysis showed how to measure the modulation in frequency bands, and how to determine the optimum attenuation. We also examined how this process changes a typical speech in noise signal.

A few additional options were presented in the final section: how fast the processing should respond to changes in the modulation, whether and how the amount of attenuation should depend on the sound pressure level, and how to combine noise reduction with WDRC.

References

ANSI. (1997). ANSI S3.5. R2002: American National Standard Methods for Calculation of the Speech Intelligibility Index. Washington, DC: American National Standards Institute.

Bentler, R., and Chiou, L.-K. (2006). Digital noise reduction: An overview. Trends in Amplification, 10(2), 67–82.

Boymans, M., and Dreschler, W.A. (2000). Field trials using a digital hearing aid with active noise reduction and dual-microphone directionality. Audiology, 39(5), 260–268.

Bray, V., and Nilsson, M.J. (2000). Objective test results support benefits of a DSP noise reduction system. The Hearing Review, 7(11), 60–65.

Bray, V., and Nilsson, M. (2001). Additive SNR benefits of signal processing features in a directional DSP aid. The Hearing Review, 8(12), 48–51, 62.

Levitt, H. (2001). Noise reduction in hearing aids: A review. Journal of Rehabilitation Research and Development, 38(1), 111–121.

Mueller, H.G., Weber, J., and Hornsby, B.W. (2006). The effects of digital noise reduction on the acceptance of background noise. Trends in Amplification, 10(2), 83–93.

Ricketts, T.A., and Hornsby, B.W. (2005). Sound quality measures for speech in noise through a commercial hearing aid implementing digital noise reduction. Journal of the American Academy of Audiology, 16(5), 270–277.

Schaub, A. (2003). Hearing Aid, United States Patent, US 6,580,798 B1, June 17.

Schaub, A. (2004). Signal processing in a hearing aid, United States Patent Application Publication, Pub. No. US 2004/0175011 A1, Sept. 9.

Schum, D.J. (2003). Noise-reduction circuitry in hearing aids: (2) Goals and current strategies. The Hearing Journal, 56(6), 32–40.

Walden, B.E., Surr, R.K., Cord, M.T., Edwards, B., and Olson, L. (2000). Comparison of benefits provided by different hearing aid technologies. Journal of the American Academy of Audiology, 11(10), 540–560.

9

Feedback Cancellation

In this chapter, we will learn how digital hearing instruments suppress the unwanted acoustic signal that feeds back from the receiver to the microphone. The analysis here will present the mainstream approach that is sometimes imprecisely referred to as phase canceling. The sections in this chapter cover

1. *A simplified model*: shows how a feedback canceller can adapt itself to a continuously changing feedback path
2. *The realistic feedback path*: presents how the simplified model extends to one that suppresses the unwanted signal arising from realistic conditions
3. *Further options*: deals with limiting the computational burden of feedback canceling and with diminishing a disturbing side effect, the phantom signal

Several studies investigated the benefit of feedback canceling and reported 10 to 15 dB feedback-margin improvement (Kuk & Ludvigsen, 2002; Greenberg et al, 2000; Dyrlund et al, 1994; Henningsen et al, 1994; Engebretson et al, 1993; Dyrlund & Bisgaard, 1991). Kates (2001) explained where the upper limit of 15 dB originates from: a feedback canceller can only cope with reflections that occur near the ear. The canceling mechanism is also useful against sub-oscillatory feedback (Latzel et al, 2001), thus supporting sound quality. For a further discussion of feedback canceling, see Parsa (2006) and Kuk et al (2002).

In practice, feedback cancellers need some circuitry in addition to the core algorithm that we will look at. This additional circuitry is beyond the scope of this book. Its purpose is to

ensure reliable operation while the instrument is processing signals of various spectral content. There are several approaches to achieve this goal, for example adaptively flattening the spectrum of control signals (Leber & Schaub, 2003), or applying frequency compression (Joson et al, 1993) to the acoustic signal.

◆ A Simplified Model

The block diagram in **Fig. 9–1** shows a simplified hearing instrument together with an external acoustic feedback path. The block diagram consists of three parts.

1. A hearing aid core – blue part
2. A feedback path that provides the route for the output signal y(t) to feed back from the receiver to microphone – green part
3. A feedback cancellation circuit that compensates for the fed-back signal – yellow part

The simplified hearing aid core processes the signal in three consecutive stages.

1. Using the band-pass filter BP, it emphasizes the signal components at frequencies around 4 kHz.
2. It then delays the signal by T = 2.5 ms, a short but realistic value for a digital hearing aid.
3. It boosts the signal by a factor of 4, that is, a 12 dB increase.

The band-pass filter is the combination of a low- and a high-pass filter that we will address

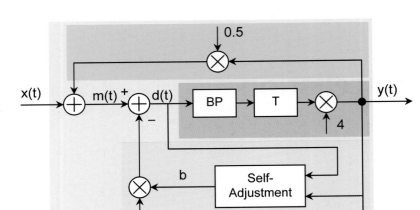

Figure 9–1   A simplified model of hearing aid and feedback path.

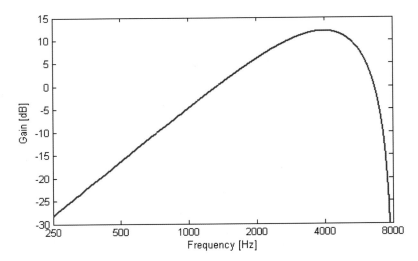

Figure 9–2   The transfer function of the hearing aid core.

in Chapter 12. **Figure 9–2** shows the transfer function resulting from the combined effects of the band-pass filter and 12-dB amplification.

The feedback path in **Fig. 9–1** simply multiplies the output signal y(t) by a factor of $^1/_2$, that is, it attenuates by 6 dB. The attenuated output signal and the input signal x(t) are added, resulting in the microphone signal m(t).

Feedback cancellation is similarly straightforward. The output signal y(t) is multiplied by factor b, and the result is then subtracted from the microphone signal m(t), producing the difference signal d(t). The self-adjustment block continuously updates factor b in response to the changing attenuation factor in the feedback path. In

this particular example, however, the attenuation in the feedback path remains at a fixed value.

As shown in the diagram, the difference signal d(t) enters the hearing aid core and passes through the three stages described above, producing the output signal y(t). In practice, the self-adjustment block then uses the signals d(t) and y(t) to continuously adjust factor b.

In our analysis, the factor b will take four different fixed values.

1. b = 0: results in no cancellation at all
2. b = 0.5: cancels the feedback
3. b = 0.25: provides insufficient suppression
4. b = 0.75: subtracts too much

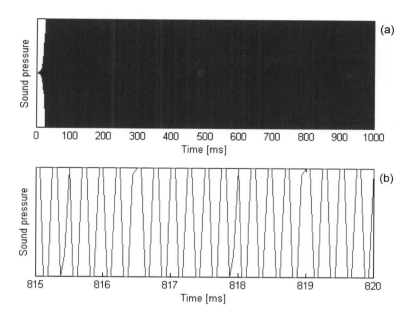

(a)

(b)

Figure 9–3 The output signal without feedback cancellation, i.e., with factor b = 0: **(a)** 1-s segment and **(b)** 5-ms segment.

Finally, by comparing the signals d(t) and y(t), it will become clear how

5. The self-adjustment block can automatically find the optimal value for factor b.

Factor b = 0

In this case, the feedback cancellation has no effect at all. It is as if the cancellation circuit was removed from the block diagram.

In the forward path the hearing aid amplifies the signal by a factor of 4, while the feedback path only attenuates the output signal by half. A signal therefore returns to the microphone with double its original sound pressure. Once the signal has passed around the loop several times, this repeated amplification causes the output signal y(t) to saturate at the hearing aid's maximum output level, producing a whistling sound.

Figure 9–3a shows that the output signal in our example reaches this maximum after only 25 ms. The 5-ms segment in **Fig. 9–3b** shows 20 periods of the output signal – corresponding exactly to 4 kHz, the frequency at which our fictitious hearing aid amplifies the signal the most.

Factor b = 0.5

This time the value of factor b corresponds exactly to the factor in the feedback path. The

feedback cancellation therefore completely cancels the fed-back signal.

Figure 9–4a shows that the input signal is the word "understand" that previously illustrated other processes throughout the book. The band-pass filter in the hearing aid core has somewhat altered the waveform shape.

Figure 9–4b shows the output signal y(t) alongside the difference signal d(t). In this example, the difference signal d(t) is identical to the input signal x(t). The nasal /n/ in the segment from 815 to 820 ms contains a low-frequency oscillation of tiny amplitude. Its period just matches the displayed 5 ms segment length; its frequency, therefore, is around 200 Hz. A higher frequency component dominates the output signal y(t) because of the band-pass filter in the hearing aid core. In the first ms, the output signal y(t) exhibits around $2^{1}/_{4}$ periods, so the frequency is around 2250 Hz.

Factor b = 0.25

Choosing an intermediate value of 0.25 for factor b brings the scheme to the verge of instability. A 4 kHz signal component, once present in the input signal, returns with twice its original amplitude to the microphone via the feedback path. The feedback canceller subtracts half of this, so that the 4 kHz signal appears in the difference signal d(t) with the same amplitude as

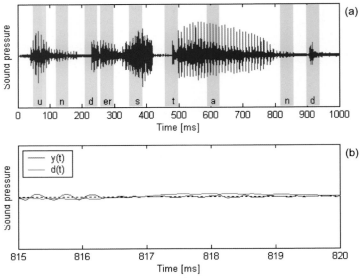

(a)

(b)

Figure 9–4   An ideal feedback cancellation with factor b = 0.5: **(a)** output signal – 1-s segment and **(b)** control signals – 5-ms segment.

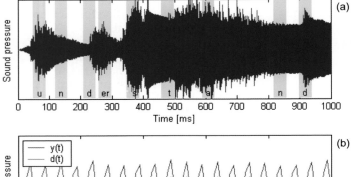

(a)

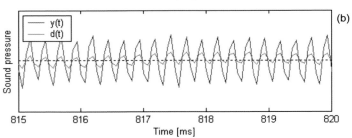

(b)

Figure 9–5   On the verge of instability with factor b = 0.25: **(a)** output signal – 1-s and **(b)** control signals – 5-ms segment.

the first time – a loop which repeats itself indefinitely.

Figure 9–5a shows the output signal. The amplitude increases as long as the 4 kHz signal component in the input signal maintains the same phase; as soon as the phase changes the feedback oscillations reduce again.

Figure 9–5b shows the relationship between the difference signal d(t) and the output signal y(t). The 4 kHz signal component appears in the

difference signal d(t) with a quarter of the amplitude that it has in the output signal y(t).

Factor b = 0.75

This case also brings the system to the verge of instability. Once a 4 kHz signal component appears in the input signal, it passes through the instrument and will feed back to the microphone with double its original amplitude. The

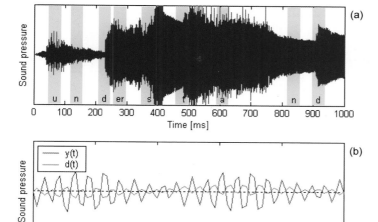

Figure 9–6 On the verge of instability with factor b = 0.75: **(a)** output signal – 1-s segment and **(b)** control signals – 5-ms segment.

feedback canceller in this case subtracts three times the original amplitude, so that the 4 kHz signal component appears in the difference signal d(t) with the same amplitude as before, but with the opposite phase.

In **Fig. 9–6a** the output signal y(t) reaches the hearing aid's maximum output level when the input signal contains a 4 kHz signal component with rapidly changing phase, such as the sibilant /s/ at 400 ms. **Figure 9–6b** again demonstrates the relationship between the difference signal d(t) and the output signal y(t). The difference signal d(t) contains the 4 kHz signal component with a quarter of the amplitude that it has in the output signal y(t), but with the opposite sign.

Self-adjustment of Factor b

The signals d(t) and y(t) serve the purpose of control signals. **Figure 9–5b** and **Fig. 9–6b** illustrate a way for the feedback canceller to find the optimum value for factor b, using a *sign rule*:

If the difference signal d(t) and the output signal y(t) have the same sign, then increase factor b by a small amount. If they are of opposite sign, reduce factor b by a similarly small amount.

In this way, factor b approaches the optimum value in tiny steps. In our example, this optimum value is 0.5; but if the value of the factor in the feedback path changes, then factor b will adapt in tiny steps, controlled by the self-adjustment mechanism.

In comparison to the simplified model, the feedback path for a real hearing instrument is more complex. We will look at this in detail in the next section. We will see how to extend the simplified model in a way that it fits the general case.

◆ The Realistic Feedback Path

When a hearing aid emits a short pulsed signal, then the microphone will detect echo signals lasting up to a few ms. This happens because the ear, head, shoulder, and nearby objects reflect the signal numerous times. Instead of a single feedback path of fixed length, the feedback canceller must account for a multitude of parallel echo paths of varying lengths. This is the basic difference compared with the simplified model of the previous section.

The block diagram in **Fig. 9–7** captures this behavior by using the symbol H(ω) to represent the feedback path. The numerous echo paths behave like a filter. They weaken the signal components of the output signal in a frequency-dependent way, and also delay them by differing amounts.

The microphone in a real hearing aid detects the sum of the sound pressures of the input

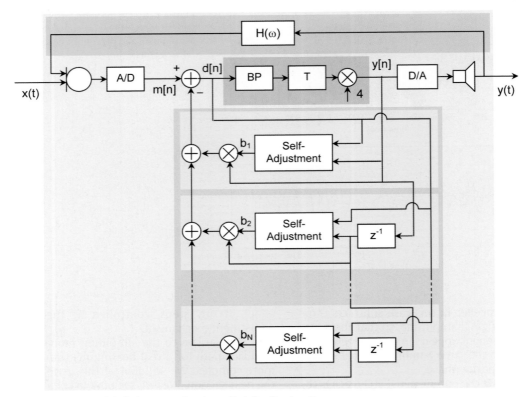

Figure 9–7   A model of a hearing aid and a realistic feedback path.

signal and the fed-back output signal. The analog-to-digital converter then samples values m[n] of the microphone signal m(t) at regular intervals. Because of the many echo paths, each sample value m[n] contains signal components of different previous values of the output signal y[n].

The yellow block in **Fig. 9–7** shows how feedback cancellation works in this case. It contains multiple copies of the feedback cancellation circuit from the simplified model in **Fig. 9–1**. From the second instance onward there is an additional block labeled z^{-1}. Each block delays the sample value at its input by one sampling interval. Consequently,

◆ The sample value y[n] multiples by factor b_1 in the first instance.

◆ The previous sample value y[n-1] multiples by factor b_2 in the second instance, and so on.

◆ Then the processing scheme sums all of these products and subtracts the sum from the sample value of the microphone signal m[n].

Two aspects determine how many instances are needed.

1. How often the hearing aid samples the signal

2. Over what time interval signal components feed back

Example: For a sampling rate of 20 kHz, N = 60 instances would be sufficient to cancel feedback signals with up to 3 ms delay.

The *sign rule* from the simplified model also extends to the feedback canceller in **Fig. 9–7**.

◆ Compare the signs of d[n] and y[n] to adjust b_1

◆ Compare the signs of d[n] and y[n-1] to adjust b_2, and so on

This processing scheme is known as an adaptive finite impulse response (FIR) filter, and the factors b_1, b_2, ..., b_N, as its filter coefficients. The filter structure is similar to the FIR filter used to implement WDRC in Chapter 5 and discussed in detail in Chapter 12, but the self-adjustment blocks here update the filter coefficients from one sampling period to the next. In their textbook, Widrow and Stearns (1985) describe a wealth of examples for the use of the adaptive FIR filter. They also discuss the quantitative aspect of setting the consecutive correction values based on the sample values of signals d[n] and y[n]. Leaving this area to the specialist literature, we instead turn to two limitations encountered when realizing and testing feedback cancellation in practice.

◆ Further Options

Clearly, feedback cancellation in its general form requires a significant amount of calculation power. In exchange for this effort, the tendency for the hearing aid to whistle diminishes. On rare occasions, however, it can itself cause an undesired signal: the phantom signal.

In this concluding section, we will determine

1. How to limit the amount of calculation power needed

2. How the *phantom signal* comes about and how to suppress it

Limiting the Computational Burden

In the example from the previous section, 60 multiplications and 60 additions are needed in each sampling interval to estimate the feedback signal, and around the same amount are needed to update the filter coefficients b_1 to b_{60}. For standard sampling, frequencies between 16 and 20 kHz are needed; this means around 2 million multiplications and additions per second.

It is therefore necessary to reduce the number of calculations wherever possible, without degrading the hearing aid performance. This is possible in the self-adjustment block. In reality, the feedback path only undergoes a significant change every now and then; for instance, when a person brings a telephone receiver to his or her ear, puts on a hat, or embraces a friend. If, on the other hand, someone just sits quietly in an armchair watching television, then the feedback path remains relatively constant. Over such lengthy intervals it is possible to update the filter coefficients less often, for example,

about a tenth as often. This mode of updating the filter coefficients is sometimes referred to as the slow-mode.

If the feedback path changes suddenly, then all of the filter coefficients need an update in every sampling interval until conditions are stable again. Only in this way is it possible to prevent the hearing aid from whistling. The feedback cancellation circuit therefore needs an additional element to identify such rapid changes. Discussing this extra element is beyond the scope of this book. However, it is important that this element only uses a small amount of processing. This is necessary for the processing scheme to preserve the savings gained from updating the filter coefficients less frequently.

Suppressing the Phantom Signal

The feedback canceller updates its filter coefficients all the time, at least in slow-mode, even when the system is in no danger of whistling due to feedback. If the input signal contains a periodic signal for a long time – for instance, the sound of a single note played on a flute – then the feedback cancellation circuit will begin to work against this signal. If the flute then stops playing the tone, the feedback canceller will continue playing it for a little while longer, and a listener will hear the *phantom signal.*

Luckily, it is quite easy to detect when this happens. If the feedback canceller is compensating for a fed-back signal, then the difference signal d[n] will be smaller than the microphone signal m[n]. If the feedback canceller generates a signal itself, however, then the level of the difference signal d[n] will exceed that of the microphone signal m[n]. In this case it makes sense to reduce all filter coefficients by large amounts at each sampling interval, until the level of the difference signal has reduced sufficiently and the *phantom signal* quickly ends.

◆ Summary

In this chapter, we established how digital hearing aids adaptively suppress the signal that feeds back from the receiver to the microphone. To this end, we investigated a simplified model of a hearing aid with an external feedback path.

The analysis showed four modes of operation, in which the simplified feedback canceller compensates not at all, too little, exactly, and too much. Building on these examples we have seen how a feedback canceller can adjust itself when the feedback path changes.

The simple model was extended to cover the general case with a realistic feedback path, which led to a review of the structure of an adaptive FIR filter. We also looked at ways to limit the computational burden. We concluded the chapter with how to suppress a *phantom signal* that occasionally arises when using a feedback canceller.

References

Dyrlund, O., and Bisgaards, N. (1991). Acoustic feedback margin improvements in hearing instruments using a prototype DFS (digital feedback suppression) system. Scandinavian Audiology, 20(1), 49–53.

Dyrlund, O., Henningsen, L.B., Bisgaard, N., and Jensen, J.H. (1994). Digital feedback suppression (DFS). Characterization of feedback-margin improvements in a DFS hearing instrument. Scandinavian Audiology, 23(2), 135–138.

Engebretson, A.M., French-St George, M., and O'Connell, M.P. (1993). Adaptive feedback stabilization of hearing aids. Scandinavian Audiology Supplement, 38, 56–64.

Greenberg, J.E., Zurek, P.M., and Brantley, M. (2000). Evaluation of feedback-reduction algorithms for hearing aids. Journal of the Acoustical Society of America, 108(5) Pt.1, 2366–2376.

Henningsen, L.B., Dyrlund, O., Bisgaard, N., and Brink, B. (1994). Digital feedback suppression (DFS). Clinical experiences when fitting a DFS hearing instrument on children. Scandinavian Audiology, 23(2), 117–122.

Joson, H.A., Asano, F., Suzuki, Y., Sone, T. (1993). Adaptive feedback cancellation with frequency compression for hearing aids. Journal of the Acoustical Society of America, 94(6), 3254–3258.

Kates, J.M. (2001). Room reverberation effects in hearing aid feedback cancellation. Journal of the Acoustical Society of America, 109(1), 367–378.

Kuk, F., and Ludvigsen, C. (2002). The real-world benefits and limitations of active digital feedback cancellation. The Hearing Review, 9(4), 64–68.

Kuk, F., Ludvigsen, C., and Kaulberg, T. (2002). Understanding feedback and digital feedback cancellation strategies. The Hearing Review, 9(2), 36–43.

Latzel, M., Gebhart, T.M., and Kiessling, J. (2001). Benefit of a digital feedback suppression system for acoustical telephone communication. Scandinavian Audiology Supplement, 52, 69–72.

Leber, R., and Schaub, A. (2003). Circuit and method for the adaptive suppression of an acoustic feedback. United States Patent US 6,611,600 B1, Aug. 26.

Parsa, V. (2006). Acoustic feedback and its reduction through digital signal processing. The Hearing Journal, 59(11), 16–23.

Widrow, B., and Stearns, S.D. (1985). Adaptive signal processing. Englewood Cliffs, NJ: Prentice Hall.

10

Sound Classification

In this chapter, we will examine how a hearing instrument identifies different acoustic environments. The more successful it is at doing this, the more reliably the hearing instrument can automatically adjust its mode of operation to fit the environment. The sections in this chapter cover

1. *Different configurations for different signal categories*: discusses sensible settings for various listening situations
2. *Periodicity*: a useful signal attribute that helps to distinguish speech, music, and noise signals from one another
3. *Spectral envelope*: another useful feature that supports sound classification
4. *Statistical evaluation*: shows how to get from signal attributes to respective categories

The intention of sound classification is to relieve the hearing-impaired person from changing programs manually or adjusting the sound intensity. The need for user controls remains, despite the high success rates of up to 95% reported in research papers (Khan et al, 2004; Lu et al, 2001; Feldbusch, 2000). In practice, sound classification works less reliably in general; a survey (Büchler, 2001) states that 75% of hearing aid users find the automatic program selection quite useful or very useful.

The analysis here just outlines this vast topic; for further details, see the review articles by Büchler et al (2005), Nordquist and Leijon (2004), and Peltonen et al (2002), and the dissertations by Nordquist (2004), Büchler (2002), and Peltonen (2001).

◆ Different Configurations for Different Signal Categories

In Chapters 5 to 9, we looked at the different signal processing blocks in digital hearing instruments. **Figure 10–1** shows, by means of a simplified block diagram, one way to combine these blocks sensibly.

At the far left of the figure, we see two microphones, the receiver is located at the far right, and in between are the different signal processing blocks.

◆ The *acoustic directionality* block processes the signals from two omnidirectional microphones and continuously generates the best directional pattern for each listening situation (as described in Chapter 7).

◆ The *noise reduction* block analyses the signal in individual frequency bands and progressively attenuates band signals, the less modulation they have (as explained in Chapter 8).

◆ The *wide dynamic range compression (WDRC)* block amplifies the signal in a frequency- and level-dependent way based on the individual hearing loss (as described in Chapters 5 and 6).

◆ The *feedback cancellation* block works to suppress the signal components that feed back from the receiver to the microphone, and adaptively adjusts itself to a changing feedback path (as explained in Chapter 9).

Next, we will look at how a hearing aid can adapt itself to the listening environment in an intelligent way, depending on the signal category: speech, music, or noise. Often more than one of

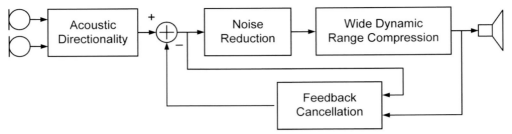

Figure 10-1   Simplified digital hearing instrument block diagram.

Table 10-1   Sensible Settings for Various Listening Situations

	Acoustic Directionality	Noise Reduction	WDRC	Feedback Cancellation
Speech	Yes, if speech is from the front	Not normally	Maximize intelligibility	Yes, if the amplification requires it
Music	Not normally, except in a reverberant room	No	Broadband amplification	No, if avoidable
Noise	Not normally	Yes, especially in case of loud noise	Depends on situation	No, if avoidable

Abbreviation: WDRC, wide dynamic range compression.

these signal types is present simultaneously, making it difficult to identify the listening situation clearly, and hence to select the appropriate processing configuration. Under these circumstances, sensible compromise values should be used. **Table 10-1** summarizes the different considerations.

Acoustic Directionality

Acoustic Directionality is beneficial in a noisy environment, where the speaker is located in front of the hearing aid wearer: for example, when two people are sitting opposite one another in a restaurant and chatting.

There are other speech situations with background noise, however, where acoustic directionality is counterproductive: for example, when driving a car and talking to a passenger or when walking together with someone along a street. In both cases, it is not possible to look at the dialog partner constantly, and a directional pattern is thus useless. It is more desirable in these cases to use an omnidirectional microphone and to switch off the hearing instrument that is farther away from the person who speaks to you.

Directionality is also generally less desirable when listening to music, except perhaps in a highly echoic room, such as a church, for example.

An omnidirectional microphone is also an advantage with many noises: wind noise, for example, and soft noises that make us aware of what is happening behind or to the side of us.

Noise Reduction

Hearing-impaired persons expect that a noise reduction system effectively attenuates loud noise.

With music, however, a noise reduction system can be distracting. The system happens to repeatedly attenuate individual band signals, or even the entire signal, as they often show only little modulation.

Noise reduction is also rather inappropriate for speech. When a system attenuates a band signal, it affects noise and speech equally and thus provides no benefit to speech intelligibility. Hearing-impaired persons usually prefer to have the whole amplified signal, even if it contains some noise.

Wide Dynamic Range Compression (WDRC)

WDRC should maximize speech intelligibility; in aiming at this objective, a fitting rationale tends to apply less gain to the low frequencies than if it pursues loudness normalization.

In contrast, broadband amplification is the best approach for music. This produces a rich sound and a feeling of proximity to the sound source.

In a noisy environment, the ideal approach depends on the exact situation. Sometimes, it is an advantage to have your attention drawn to the noises around you, while at other times they are simply annoying.

Feedback Cancellation

Feedback cancellation is at its most useful when the hearing aid provides a lot of mid- and high-frequency gain, such as to optimize speech intelligibility.

In other listening situations, such as listening to music for example, the hearing aid may apply less gain at these frequencies, and the feedback canceller could generally be disabled. This has two advantages: it reduces the power consumption, and prevents the rare phantom signal effect, as described in Chapter 9.

◆ Periodicity

Acoustic signals can be analyzed to see whether they are periodic. If they are, how often their sound pressure oscillations repeat within a short time period can also be determined.

Music signals are generally periodic in nature, whereas most noise signals are aperiodic. Speech contains a mix, changing constantly between voiced and unvoiced phonemes; the voiced phonemes are periodic, the unvoiced ones are not.

The first glance at a short signal segment will reveal whether or not it is periodic. The length of the individual period is also immediately obvious. Let us look at short segments taken from the word "understand" introduced in Chapter 1. **Figure 10–2** shows 40-ms segments of the nasal sound /n/, the sibilant /s/ and the vowel sound /æ/.

◆ The nasal sound /n/ in **Fig. 10–2a** is clearly periodic. The sound pressure oscillations repeat themselves with a gap of 8.5 ms, namely, with a fundamental frequency of ~120 Hz. Interleaving yellow and white background marks the periods within the waveform.

◆ The waveform for the sibilant /s/ in **Fig. 10–2b**, on the other hand, is aperiodic.

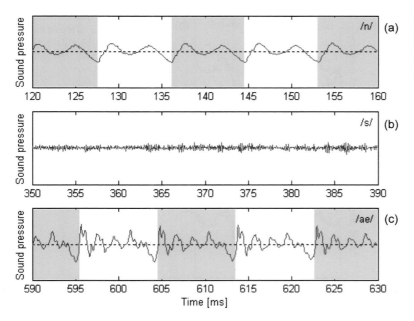

Figure 10–2 Waveform of various phonemes taken from the word "understand": **(a)** nasal sound /n/, **(b)** sibilant /s/, and **(c)** vowel sound /æ/.

◆ The vowel sound /æ/ in **Fig. 10–2c** is again periodic, with a period of almost 10 ms, namely, with a fundamental frequency of around 100 Hz.

What is easy for us to see translates into a huge arithmetic task for the processor in the digital hearing instrument. To identify whether a signal is periodic, the processor must first calculate the *autocorrelation*, or more precisely, the autocorrelation coefficient. In Chapter 14, I will present the calculation details; here we will establish how this characteristic helps to distinguish different types of signal from one another.

Autocorrelation is concerned with how well a short signal segment matches a previous segment from the same signal. The autocorrelation coefficient quantifies the amount of correspondence between the current and old segments, taking values between −1 and +1.

A value close to +1 indicates that the waveforms in the two segments mostly match. If the value is around 0, then the signals are completely different. A value of close to −1 indicates that the waveforms are almost identical, but of opposite phase, with inverse sign.

Figure 10–3 illustrates, by means of an example showing the nasal sound /n/, how the autocorrelation coefficient takes positive and negative values. The diagrams all show the same 20-ms signal segment from **Fig. 10–2a** displayed as a blue curve, and they each show a time-delayed signal segment in green:

◆ **Figure 10–3a**: with a time delay of $\Delta T = 2$ ms the signals end up with opposite phase, and the autocorrelation coefficient becomes negative, $r = -0.8$.

◆ **Figure 10–3b**: the segments are delayed by $\Delta T = 4$ ms with respect to one another, so by around half a period. By chance, this results in a similar waveform, with an autocorrelation coefficient of $r = 0.6$.

◆ **Figure 10–3c**: when the time difference is $\Delta T = 6$ ms, the signals again end up with opposite phase, resulting in an autocorrelation coefficient of $r = -0.7$.

◆ **Figure 10–3d**: a time delay of $\Delta T = 8$ ms, in other words practically an entire period, ends up with almost a total match between signal segments. As a result, the autocorrelation coefficient is $r = 0.7$ and it increases further to 0.99, when an additional 0.5-ms delay makes the signals match completely.

Next, we will examine the everyday signals from Chapter 1, using the color code in **Fig. 10–4** to represent the value of the autocorrelation. We will first look at speech, and then go on to music, pulsed noise, and monotonic noise.

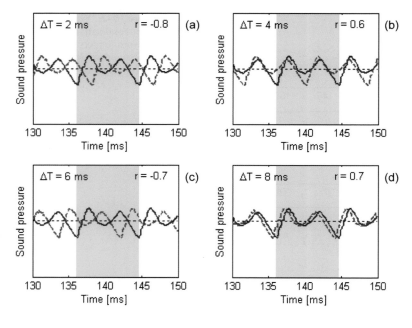

Figure 10–3 Autocorrelation coefficient r for different time delays ΔT: **(a)** $\Delta T = 2$ ms, **(b)** $\Delta T = 4$ ms, **(c)** $\Delta T = 6$ ms, and **(d)** $\Delta T = 8$ ms.

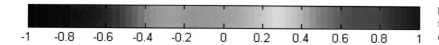

Figure 10–4   Color code for autocorrelation coefficients.

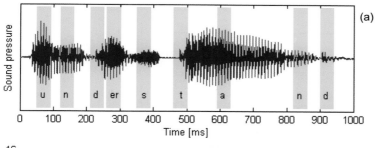

(a)

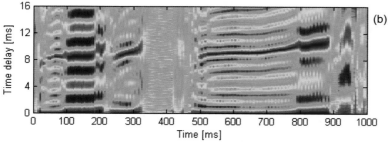

(b)

Figure 10–5   The word "understand": (a) waveform and (b) autocorrelation coefficient.

Speech

Figure 10–5 shows the first example, the waveform of the word "understand" in **Fig. 10–5a** and the autocorrelation coefficient in **Fig. 10–5b**. Unlike a spectrogram that shows frequency on the y-axis, **Fig. 10-5b** shows the delay between signal segments on the y-axis, with a range of 0 to 16 ms.

The change between periodic and aperiodic intervals is typical for speech. In **Fig. 10–5b**, the dark red region in the first 330 ms indicates the periodicity of the phonemes in the first two syllables. As we see from the y-axis, the period has values between 8 and 10 ms, which corresponds to a fundamental frequency of between 100 and 125 Hz.

The following interval, of up to around 410 ms, contains the aperiodic waveform of the sibilant /s/. **Figure 10–5b** uses the colors light blue to yellow to represent the accordingly low autocorrelation coefficient values of between −0.2 and +0.2.

The dark red region from around 510 ms on to 890 ms indicates the periodicity of the phonemes /æ/ and /n/. The period increases from around 9 ms to over 10 ms, so the funda-

mental frequency decreases accordingly, from ~110 Hz to below 100 Hz. This is also typical speech behavior: the fundamental frequency changes slowly according to the speech melody.

Music

Autocorrelation gives completely different pictures for different signals. The piece of easy listening music for flute and guitar makes this clear: **Fig. 10–6a** shows its waveform and **Fig. 10–6b** the autocorrelation coefficient.

This piece of music fits the statement about musical signals made at the beginning of this section. The signal is periodic throughout the entire 6-s segment. And, in contrast to speech, the period – and with it the fundamental frequency – is constant over successive time intervals, as one would expect from a sequence of tones.

The period of the first tone is slightly above 10 ms, with a frequency of just less than 100 Hz. Then five more tones, increasing in frequency, follow within the first 2 s; their periods accordingly decrease from around 5 ms down to around 2 ms.

The diagram shows a regular striped pattern. How does this happen? For the tone with the

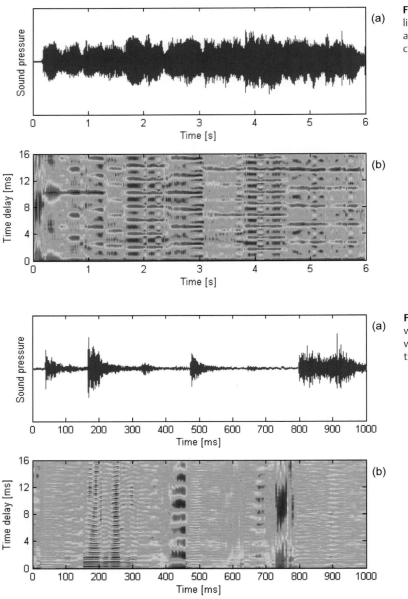

Figure 10–6 A piece of easy listening music: **(a)** waveform and **(b)** autocorrelation coefficient.

Figure 10–7 Noise made when doing the dishes: **(a)** waveform and **(b)** autocorrelation coefficient.

2 ms period, for example, the autocorrelation coefficient gets close to $+1$, when comparing the current signal segment with one that lies back in time by 2 ms. Due to the periodicity, the autocorrelation coefficient again gets close to $+1$, when comparing the current signal segment with one that lies back in time by an integer multiple of 2 ms (i.e., by 4, 6, 8, 10, 12, 14 ms, etc.). This is how the striped pattern comes about.

As noted before, music typically has this kind of continuous periodicity, where the signal has one period for a certain time before abruptly changing to a different period. This attribute constitutes an interesting clue for a hearing instrument to turn off the noise reduction, even if the signal only contains minimal modulation.

Pulsed Noise

Next, in **Fig. 10–7a**, we see an example of the pulsed noise made by clattering crockery and cutlery together when doing the dishes.

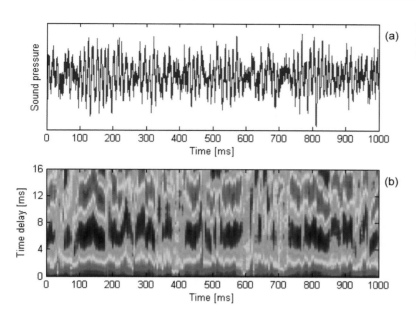

Figure 10–8 Monotonic train noise: **(a)** waveform and **(b)** autocorrelation coefficient.

The autocorrelation coefficient in **Fig. 10–7b** again appears quite different to the previous examples.

In this case, the autocorrelation coefficient consists predominantly of low values, around 0, as evidenced by the colors in the range between light blue and yellow. Short periodic segments occur randomly, for instance, between 400 and 450 ms, and again between 650 and 700 ms. The periods are around 4 ms in the first instance, and 2 ms in the second.

Two other periodic segments stand out, where the periods take extreme values. Between 150 and 300 ms, the period is clearly less than 1 ms; between 700 and 800 ms, it exceeds 15 ms.

This extremely irregular behavior clearly distinguishes the signal from both speech and music. Hence, it is another clue for a hearing instrument to effectively attenuate pulsed noise, despite its considerable modulation.

Monotonic Noise

Next, let us look at another signal that falls into the noise category, the monotonic sound of a train, shown in **Fig. 10–8a**. As we have seen in Chapter 1, the train noise has only minimal modulation over the entire frequency range. As a result, conventional noise reduction works well with this type of noise.

The monotonic noise is strictly aperiodic. Nevertheless, the autocorrelation coefficient

in **Fig. 10–8b** is consistently high in value, and lies almost continuously around 0.9. At the same time, the value of this apparent period changes quickly and irregularly between 10 and 16 ms, which corresponds to a fast changing fundamental frequency between 60 and 100 Hz. This low and unstable fundamental frequency is typical of low frequency noise, and distinguishes it well from the other signal categories.

These examples show that periodicity helps to distinguish between the different signal categories. It works even better if the processor evaluates further signal attributes, such as the spectral envelope, for example.

◆ Spectral Envelope

Let us first make clear what the term *spectral envelope* means. The black dotted line in **Fig. 10–9a** shows the spectrum of the sibilant /s/ and in **Fig. 10–9b** the spectrum of the vowel sound /æ/ in the word "understand."

The diagrams each contain three additional solid curves. These so-called envelopes describe the coarse trend of the spectrum, as follows:

◆ Blue – first-order envelope, based on a single parameter. This shows how steeply the overall spectrum slopes; for the sibilant /s/ it increases

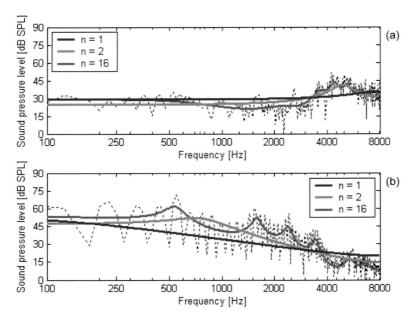

Figure 10–9   Spectrum and spectral envelopes of phonemes from the word "understand": **(a)** sibilant /s/ and **(b)** vowel sound /æ/.

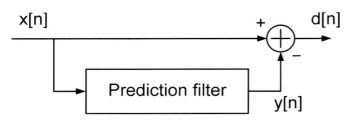

Figure 10–10   Evaluation of the prediction error.

slightly, and for the vowel sound /æ/ it drops conspicuously toward the high frequencies.

◆ Green – second-order envelope, based on two parameters. This reproduces a single resonance – the dominant one; for the sibilant /s/ it is only slightly pronounced, for the vowel sound /æ/ it is more so.

◆ Red – sixteenth-order envelope, based on 16 parameters. Of the examples, this most closely approximates the spectrum, sticking close to the peaks of the oscillating curve and including up to eight resonances.

The diagrams make it clear: the higher the order, the more closely the envelope will resemble the spectrum. This added precision is, however, only won at an increasing computational burden for the hearing instrument. It is therefore good to know that the spectra of vari-

ous sounds differ even in their gross shape, that is, in their low-order envelopes.

In chapter 15, numerical examples will show

◆ How to calculate the envelope parameters for a given signal segment

◆ How the single parameter of a first-order envelope defines the gradient of a spectrum

◆ How the two parameters of a second-order envelope define its dominant resonance

The analysis here focuses on a more fundamental, underlying aspect: *predictability*. **Figure 10–10** introduces the concept. An input signal $x[n]$ passes through a prediction filter. This filter calculates an estimate, $y[n]$, of the current signal value, $x[n]$, based on the preceding input samples, $x[n-1]$, $x[n-2]$, etc. The difference between the real signal value $x[n]$ and the estimate $y[n]$ gives the difference signal $d[n]$.

If the input signal consists of white noise, with a flat spectrum, then any attempt will fail to predict the current value based on previous ones. The more pronounced the slope present in a signal's spectrum – or the more marked the resonances – the better the prediction will work. The opposite extreme to white noise is a pure tone featuring a single spectral line; its waveform can be predicted exactly. Note, however, that the analysis here is not about predicting a waveform due to periodicity, but with respect to a time span that, in general, is much shorter than a signal's period.

If the prediction filter is able to generate good estimates for a signal $x[n]$, the difference signal $d[n]$ will consist of smaller sample values than the input signal $x[n]$. A readily calculable quantity captures how well the prediction works: the *normalized prediction error*. This quantity is defined as the ratio of two sums of squares: the sum of squares of the difference samples $d[n]$ divided by sum of squares of the input samples $x[n]$. To determine the normalized prediction error thus requires carrying out the following three steps:

1. Square the difference samples $d[n]$ and sum up the squared values

2. Square the input samples $x[n]$ and sum up the squared values

3. Divide the first sum by the second

The normalized prediction error complies with the following rule:

The nearer its value is to 1, the flatter the spectrum of the analyzed signal; and on the other hand, the closer it is to 0, the steeper is the rise or fall in the spectrum, or the more pronounced are its resonances.

In addition to the items above, the numerical examples in Chapter 15 will reveal two more features.

1. How the spectral envelope and the prediction filter interrelate

2. How it is possible to calculate the normalized prediction error directly from the envelope parameters

Let us now focus on how the normalized prediction error helps to distinguish different signals from one another. We will first look at speech, and then go on to music, pulsed noise, and monotonic noise.

Speech

Figure 10–11a shows the waveform of the word "understand." The various phonemes clearly differ in their normalized prediction error, as **Fig. 10–11b** shows. The diagram contains a blue and a green curve to represent the results for first- and second-order prediction, respectively. The curves reveal the following key points:

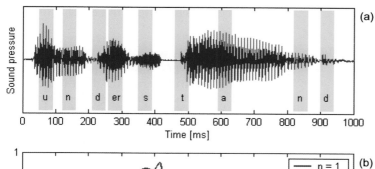

(a)

Figure 10–11 The word "understand": **(a)** waveform and **(b)** normalized prediction error.

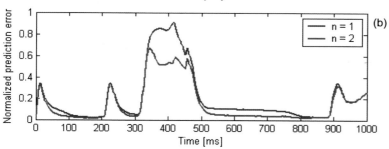

(b)

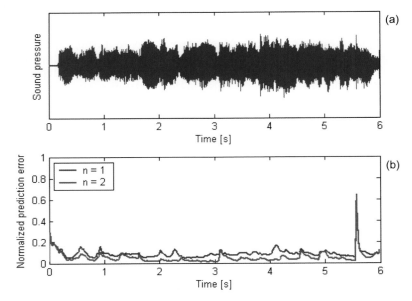

(a)

(b)

Figure 10–12   A piece of easy listening music: **(a)** waveform and **(b)** normalized prediction error.

◆ Sibilant /s/: the part of the blue curve representing the /s/ has the value 0.9, which means the spectrum is slightly tilted; the corresponding part of the green curve is at 0.5, so it has a slightly pronounced resonance, as previously seen in **Fig. 10–9a**.

◆ Vowel sound /æ/: the blue curve is at 0.1, therefore it has a significant spectral gradient; the corresponding green curve has a value of 0.05, which indicates the presence of an additional dominant resonance, as previously seen in **Fig. 10–9b**.

◆ Nasal sound /n/: both curves are at 0.05, so it has a very steeply sloping spectrum.

◆ Stop consonant /d/: both curves have the value 0.35; therefore it has only a moderately steep spectrum without any significant resonance.

Music

Next, we will look at the extract of easy listening music for flute and guitar in **Fig. 10–12a**. The curves in **Fig. 10–12b** have values of below 0.2 for almost the entire segment. This implies a spectrum with a substantial gradient. The spectrum also contains a dominant resonance because the green curve lies mostly below the blue one, indicating that the second-order prediction filter produces a lower prediction error than the

first-order filter. In all, the prediction errors behave in a similar way to the vowels in a speech signal, although music sounds quite different than speech.

The recording contains an anomaly toward the end of the time segment. The normalized prediction error increases for a moment, to a value of 0.6. What is happening? When you play the guitar you constantly change the chord grip, and occasionally strum the strings. This produces an audible sound. The normalized prediction error is reacting to this effect at time 5.6 s.

Pulsed Noise

Figure 10–13a shows the waveform that results from clattering the dishes. The normalized prediction error in **Fig. 10–13b** again covers a large range of values. When plates and cutlery clatter together the values lie between 0.6 and 0.9. The spectrum is therefore slightly tilted, and at the same time slightly curved, as indicated by the green curve's lower values. Only when the clattering dies down, does the value tend to go toward 0.2 or lower. This low value, in turn, points to a light background noise with a substantial spectral gradient.

So, not only the periodicity, but also the normalized prediction error differs significantly between our example of pulsed noise and speech, in contrast to modulation, which is pro-

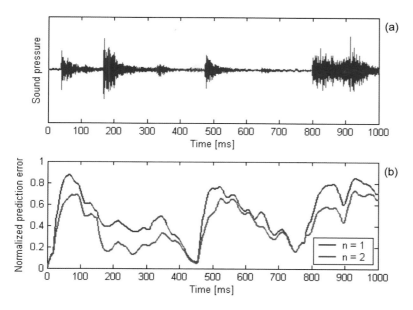

Figure 10–13 Noise made when doing the dishes: **(a)** waveform and **(b)** normalized prediction error.

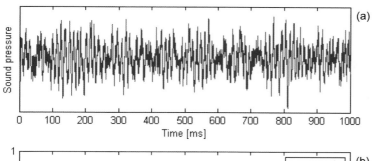

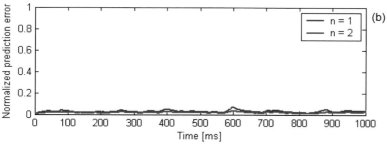

Figure 10–14 Monotonic train noise: **(a)** waveform and **(b)** normalized prediction error.

nounced for both signal types. Hence, the normalized prediction error constitutes another clue for a hearing aid to apply noise reduction to the pulsed noise, despite its high modulation.

Monotonic Noise

As a final example in **Fig. 10–14a,** we will look again at the monotonic noise generated by a train passing through a tunnel. In this case, the spectrum has such an extreme gradient that the normalized prediction error in **Fig. 10–14b** consistently lies below 0.05, even with the first-order prediction filter.

The prediction error in this example does not tell us much else, except perhaps that it is a little less suited to distinguishing noise from music – compare **Fig. 10–14b** with **Fig. 10–12b** to this end. However, it is typical for signal attributes to occasionally provide vague information. This thought naturally leads to the topic of the next section.

◆ Statistical Evaluation

Once sufficient signal attributes are calculated, the first step is complete. The previous two sections just presented a few examples: *periodicity* along with *fundamental frequency,* and *spectral gradient* along with *dominant resonance.* These attributes complement *sound pressure level* and *modulation* that we looked at in previous chapters.

However, just as the short time variations in sound pressure level create the additional attribute *modulation,* so too the attributes introduced in this chapter may generate further useful attributes. The short-time variation of the fundamental frequency is an example. Additional questions then present themselves: Does this new attribute change in jumps or continuously? If continuously, how fast does it change?

Which attributes are best, and how many are actually needed, remains a research topic. Here we turn to the question of what is necessary for a hearing aid to allocate a signal to one of the signal categories. There are two distinct tasks:

1. *Compile a statistical basis:* determine in advance how often each attribute takes what values, split by signal category, for as comprehensive a sample set as possible, preferably with a sample set that takes the individual listening environment into account. For this reason, modern fitting software is programmed to ask questions about personal lifestyle or predominant listening situations.

2. *Categorize the acoustic signal*: constantly calculate the continuous attributes in the current signal and allocate the signal to the appropriate category—to that with attribute values closest to those calculated from the signal.

Several factors make the statistical basis complicated; there is a great number of signal attributes and they differ in format. For example, the sound pressure level takes values from a continuous range, whereas the periodicity attribute simply takes one of two possible values, periodic or aperiodic. Furthermore, a fundamental frequency is only sometimes present.

Luckily, it is possible to clarify the statistical background by means of a relatively simple example; and for a thorough discussion, see Gatti (2005) or Pestman (1998). Assume that you know only two attributes about a student at a German university, height and body mass index (BMI). Based on this, you should guess whether the student is male or female.

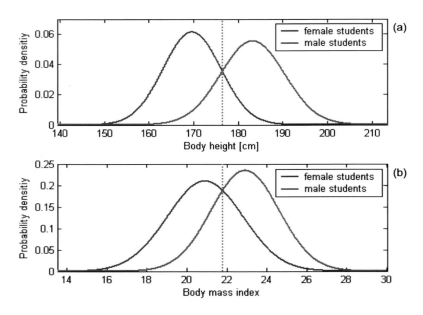

Figure 10–15　Examples of statistical distributions: **(a)** body height and **(b)** body mass index.

So, instead of the three signal categories *speech*, *music*, and *noise*, in this simple example there are just two categories: *male students* and *female students*. There are also only two attributes: *height* and *BMI*.

The goal of the first step is to lay the statistical foundation. **Figure 10–15a** shows how often different heights occur for the students, separated by gender. The curves exhibit the typical shape of a normal distribution: Gaussian bell curves, named after the German mathematician Johann Carl Friedrich Gauss. The diagram shows that the most common height for female students is 169 cm (5'6.5"), and for male students it is 183 cm (6').

The BMI tells us whether a person is over- or underweight without needing to know weight and height simultaneously. The body mass index can be calculated using the formula:

$$BMI = (body\ weight[kg])/$$
$$(height[m])^2 \qquad \text{(Eq. 10-1)}$$

Figure 10–15b shows which BMI values occur and how often, again separated by gender. The most common value for female students is 20.9, and for male students it is 22.9.

How is it possible to make a decision based on a given height? A red dotted line in **Fig. 10–15a** marks the threshold value of 176 cm: larger values occur more often for male students than for female students. If the height exceeds this threshold, then one would suspect a male student; and if it is below, one would guess a female student.

Of course, there are also taller women and shorter men; there will therefore be some incorrect decisions based solely on height. We see this in **Fig. 10–15a** where the distributions overlap. Using this diagram it is possible to estimate the risk of thinking that a female student is a man. It is 15% and is equivalent to the area under the blue curve to the right of the threshold value, when compared with the total area under the entire blue curve. At 17% the risk is slightly greater that a male student could be mistaken for a woman.

It is similar for the acoustic signals: each of the attributes also follows a distribution function, and these distribution functions for different signal categories also overlap. So in this case too, it is possible to make a decision by weighing up which signal category is most likely. And the result will sometimes be wrong too.

However, back to our simple example: **Fig. 10–15b** shows that the BMI distribution functions overlap even more significantly than those for the height. The probability of error here is significantly greater, with values of 32% and 25%.

The picture gets quite different when the decision is based on both attributes at the same time. **Figure 10–16** shows the statistical background.

In **Fig. 10–16a,** we see the normal distributions for male and female students: Gaussian bells plotted against the axes *body height* and *BMI*. A combination of height and BMI corresponds to a point on the area spanned by the two axes, and the normal distributions then define how often this combination occurs for male and female students, respectively. The distribution with the larger value at a given point determines if a student with a given height and BMI is more likely to be male or female.

Figure 10–16b comprises an upper and a lower level. On the lower level, curves with equal probability are displayed – similar to contour lines on a map. On the upper level, the area is divided into two regions. One of them represents the region where the combination of BMI and height is more common for female students, and the other where the combination is more common for male students.

By using both attributes together, the decision-making is more reliable. The reason for this is that the two-dimensional normal distributions end up farther apart on the area than their projection profiles in **Figs. 10–15a** and **10–15b**. This means they overlap less, and the risk of making the wrong choice is reduced. In our example this error rate is now 7% and is the same for errors in either direction.

The success rate also improves for the acoustic signals when the decisions are based on more attributes. However, with an increasing number of attributes it becomes more difficult to divide the space into easily computable sections assigned to the different signal categories. New mathematical techniques, such as neural networks, are in use for these applications. The theory of neural networks exceeds the scope of this book; for a thorough discussion, see Dreyfus (2005), Rojas and Feldman (1996), or Strickland et al (1995).

The new techniques render it unnecessary to determine the distribution functions for the

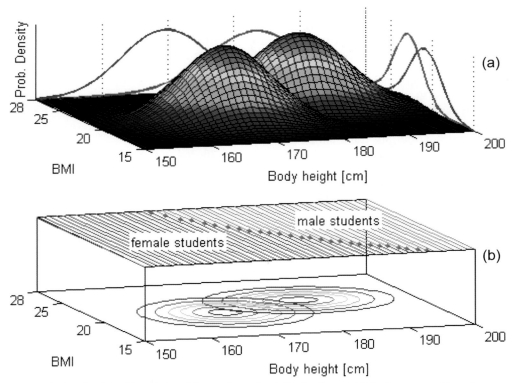

Figure 10–16   Statistical foundation: **(a)** two-dimensional distributions and **(b)** category-specific regions and contours of equal probability.

signal attributes; instead it is now necessary to train the neural network. To a certain degree, a neural network can be compared with an adaptive filter as discussed in Chapter 9. The arithmetic procedure is predetermined, and entails the correct adjustment of a large number of coefficients, in such a way that the neural network later allocates the real signal to the correct category. Training the network again requires a comprehensive sample of acoustic signals of known categories. The coefficients are then adjusted with the large number of samples, by repeatedly taking small steps in the right direction.

how to configure the various signal processing blocks in a hearing aid to optimize the processing of different signals.

New signal attributes were presented: periodicity along with fundamental frequency, and gradient of the spectrum along with dominant resonance. The analysis focused on how well the attributes distinguish between example signals of different categories.

Finally, we established how to evaluate the signal attributes. This process involves statistical techniques that make it possible to categorize a signal correctly most of the time; nevertheless, there is always a risk that a decision will be wrong.

◆ Summary

In this chapter, we dealt with the way a hearing aid automatically adapts itself to different listening situations. To this end, we determined

References

Büchler, M. (2001). How good are automatic program selection features? The Hearing Review, 8(9), 50–54, 84.

Büchler, M. (2002). Algorithms for sound classification in hearing instruments. Doctoral dissertation, Swiss Federal Institute of Technology, Zurich, Switzerland.

———. How good are automatic program selection features? The Hearing Review, 8(9), 50–54, 84.

Büchler, M., Allegro, S., Launer, S., and Dillier, N. (2005). Sound classification in hearing aids inspired by auditory scene analysis, EURASIP. Journal on Applied Signal Processing, 18, 2991–3002.

Dreyfus, G. (2005). Neural networks: Methodology and applications. New York/Heidelberg/Berlin: Springer.

Feldbusch, F. (2000). Identification of Noises by Neural Nets for Application in Hearing Aids. Paper presented at the 2nd International Symposium on Neural Computation, Berlin, Germany.

Gatti, P. L. (2005). Probability theory and mathematical statistics for engineers. London, UK: Spon Press.

Khan, M. K. S., Al-Khatib, W. G., and Moinuddin, M. (2004). Automatic classification of speech and music using neural networks. Paper presented the Second ACM International Workshop on Multimedia Databases, Arlington, VA.

Lu, L., Jiang, H., and Zhang, H. J. (2001). A robust audio classification and segmentation method. Paper presented at the 9th ACM International Conference on Multimedia, Ottawa, Canada.

Nordquist, P. (2004). Sound classification in hearing instruments. Doctoral dissertation, Royal Institute of Technology, Stockholm, Sweden.

Nordqvist, P., and Leijon, A. (2004). An efficient robust sound classification algorithm for hearing aids. The Journal of the Acoustical Society of America, 115(6), 3033–3041.

Peltonen, V. (2001). Computational auditory scene recognition. Master's thesis, University of Technology, Tampere, Finland.

Peltonen, V., Tuomi, J., Klapuri, A., Huopaniemi, J., and Sorsa, T. (2002). Computational auditory scene recognition. Paper presented at the International Conference on Acoustics, Speech, and Signal Processing, Orlando, FL.

Pestman, W.R. (1998): Mathematical statistics: An introduction. Berlin: Walter de Gruyter.

Rojas, R., and Feldman, J. (1996). Neural networks: A systematic introduction. New York/Heidelberg/Berlin: Springer.

Strickland, M. T., Reinhardt J., and Müller, B. (1995). Neural networks: An introduction. New York/Heidelberg/Berlin: Springer.

Part III

Calculations in the Digital Processor

11

Segment-wise Processing with Fourier Transforms

In this chapter, an overview is given of the Fourier transform and its use in processing digitized signals, also termed *discrete* signals. Today's computers and processors use a particularly efficient version of the *discrete Fourier transform*, named the *fast Fourier transform* (FFT). Amazingly, this algorithm celebrates its 200-year jubilee: Carl Friedrich Gauss discovered it around 1805, as was documented later (Gauss, 1866). In the last century, Cooley and Tukey (1965) independently rediscovered the algorithm and paved the way for its use in digital signal processing.

The FFT technique allows modifying signal components at different frequencies independently of each other. It thus lends itself to all kinds of signal processing, from compression limiting to wide dynamic range compression (WDRC), as well as noise reduction and more. The sections in this chapter cover

1. *Transformation into the frequency domain*: illustrates by examples what result the Fourier transform produces

2. *Processing a single signal segment*: shows how to modify a signal segment by transforming it into the frequency domain, changing its spectrum, and finally transforming the altered spectrum back into a signal segment in the time-domain

3. *Processing a continuous signal in consecutive segments*: extends the procedure from the previous section to process a continuous signal as a series of overlapping signal segments

The analysis here will focus on a graphic description; for a purely mathematical presentation, see Butz (2005), Beerends et al (2003), or Walker (1996).

◆ Transformation into the Frequency Domain

We will look at a few sample signals to see how the Fourier transform works. **Figure 11–1a** shows four periods of a cosine signal, that is a harmonic oscillation with a sample value of 1 at time 0.

Figure 11–1b illustrates the result of a discrete Fourier transform. The x-axis shows frequencies with index values from 0 to 64. At index value 4 there is a vertical line upward with an amplitude of 1 – due to the four periods in the segment. At all other frequency indices the amplitude is 0.

Next, **Fig. 11–2a** shows the harmonic oscillation, when delayed such that it produces a sine signal with a sample value of 0 at time 0; **Fig. 11–2b** shows its spectrum. There is again an amplitude of 1 at frequency index 4, but this time the amplitude points out along the horizontal coordinate axis.

There is a rule to this effect:

The amplitude appears in the frequency domain like a hand on a clock face. The length of the hand remains unchanged, as long as the waveform amplitude is the same; and the orientation of the hand shows the phase of the signal.

Figure 11–3a shows a harmonic oscillation with additional delay. Furthermore, the amplitude is halved, and the frequency is doubled, so

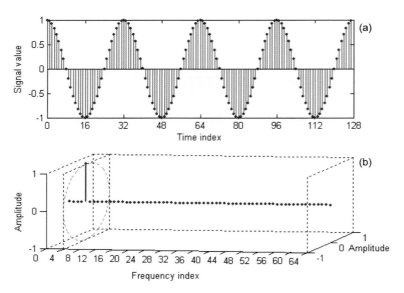

Figure 11–1   The Fourier transform of a cosine signal: **(a)** waveform and **(b)** spectrum.

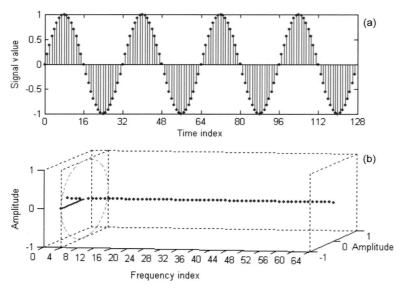

Figure 11–2   The Fourier transform of a sine signal: **(a)** waveform and **(b)** spectrum.

there are eight periods within the time segment. The spectrum in **Fig. 11–3b** shows an amplitude of 0.5 pointing vertically down, at the frequency index 8.

Having seen how the Fourier transform acts on simple sinusoidal signals, we will now turn to its use for processing slightly more complex signals.

◆ **Processing a Single Signal Segment**

In this and the next section a sample signal is used that is composed of two harmonic oscillations. Their frequencies are such that the waveforms in **Figs. 11–4** contain 4 and 32 periods, respectively.

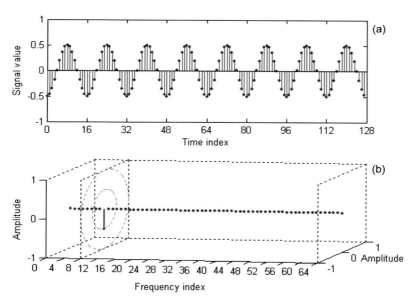

Figure 11–3 The Fourier transform of an inverted cosine signal: **(a)** waveform and **(b)** spectrum.

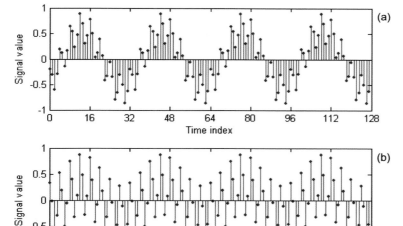

Figure 11–4 The sum of harmonic oscillations with differing amplitudes: **(a)** predominant low-frequency component and **(b)** predominant high-frequency component.

The low-frequency oscillation has an amplitude of 0.6 in **Fig. 11–4a**, and the high-frequency oscillation has an amplitude of 0.3. In **Fig. 11–4b** the amplitude values are exchanged.

We can consider the signal in **Fig. 11–4a** to be the input signal to a processing system, and the signal in **Fig. 11–4b** the output signal that the system provides by halving the amplitude of the low-frequency oscillation, and doubling that of the high-frequency part.

Figure 11–5a shows the spectrum of the signal in **Fig. 11–4a**, and **Fig. 11–5b** shows the spectrum of the signal in **Fig. 11–4b**. Let us now consider how to transform the input signal into the output signal using the following three processing steps:

1. Apply the Fourier transform to the signal segment to get its spectrum: this step takes us from **Fig. 11–4a** to **Fig. 11–5a**. The spectrum

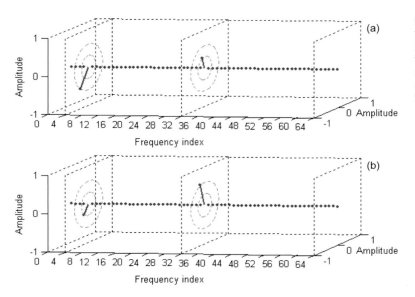

Figure 11–5 The Fourier transform of the sum of harmonic oscillations with differing amplitudes: **(a)** predominant low-frequency component and **(b)** predominant high-frequency component.

confirms that the amplitudes are 0.6 and 0.3 at frequency indices 4 and 32, respectively, and 0 at all other frequency indices.

2. Change the amplitudes in the spectrum by applying desired multiplication factors: in our example, this step involves halving the amplitude at index 4 and doubling that at index 32, thus taking us from **Fig. 11–5a** to **Fig. 11–5b**.

3. Apply an inverse Fourier transform to the spectrum to get the waveform in the time domain: the *inverse* Fourier transform performs the opposite operation to the Fourier transform; in our example, it transforms the spectrum from **Fig. 11–5b** into its corresponding time domain waveform in **Fig. 11–4b**.

We may think of the inverse Fourier transform as a kind of synthesizer that generates all the harmonics contained in a spectrum—whereas the Fourier transform is the analysis tool that detects all the harmonics present in a waveform.

Next, we will look at how to extend the three-step procedure to a realistic case for processing a continuous signal instead of an isolated segment only.

◆ Processing a Continuous Signal in Consecutive Segments

From the instant that a hearing instrument is switched on, it must continuously process the acoustic signal. The procedure described in the previous section only addresses discrete segments. So, to use the procedure in a hearing aid, the continuous signal must first be broken up into consecutive segments—into overlapping segments, actually—to ensure smooth transitions. Textbooks on time-frequency signal processing explore this subject in detail; see Papandreou (2003) or Zölzer et al (2002).

This section will use the same sample signal as the previous one, but will start with the analog signal representation. As a result, the diagrams will label the time-axis with ms (millisecond) and the frequency-axis with Hz (Hertz).

Figure 11–6a shows the analog input signal over a 16-ms time interval, containing eight periods of the low-frequency oscillation. **Figures 11–6b–11–6d** show the input signal after analog-to-digital (A/D) conversion, split into three overlapping segments of 8-ms duration each. Every segment consists of 128 samples as in the previous example. The signal is faded in at the start of each segment and faded out at the end, so that the signal runs smoothly at the segment boundaries.

Next, the procedure described in the previous section goes into action. **Figure 11–7a** illustrates the spectrum of one of the three signal segments. The diagram shows small additional amplitudes adjacent to the main ones at frequencies 500 Hz and 4 kHz, corresponding to the frequency indices 4 and 32. These additional amplitudes are due to fading the signal in and out. However, they

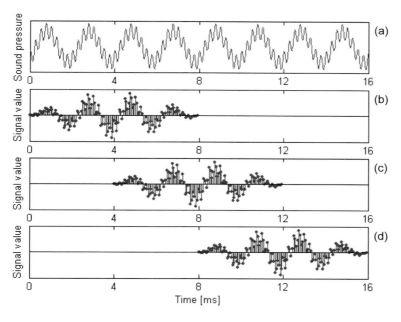

Figure 11–6 Splitting a signal into overlapping segments: **(a)** continuous signal, **(b)** first segment, **(c)** second segment, and **(d)** third segment.

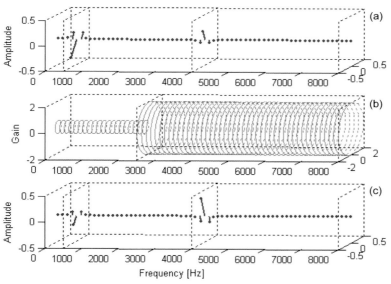

Figure 11–7 Processing a segment in the frequency domain: **(a)** spectrum of input signal, **(b)** gain, and **(c)** spectrum of output signal.

do not have an impact on the reconstructed waveform in the time domain, as we will see shortly.

Figure 11–7b illustrates the desired amplification: double the amplitude of all signal components above 2.5 kHz, and halve the amplitude of all signal components at lower frequencies. By applying this operation to the amplitudes in **Fig. 11–7a,** the spectrum of the desired output signal is produced, as shown in **Fig. 11–7c.**

The last step transforms from the frequency domain into the time domain. The procedure again fades in the start of each segment, and fades out the end. In this way, it generates the signals shown in **Figs. 11–8a—11–8c.** Adding these partial signals together and passing them through a digital-to-analog (D/A) converter finally produces the analog output signal shown in **Fig. 11–8d.**

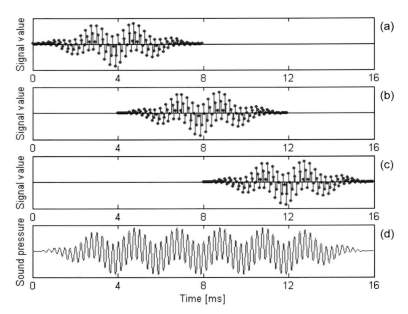

Figure 11–8 Combination of processed signals into an output signal: **(a)** first segment, **(b)** second segment, **(c)** third segment, and **(d)** continuous signal.

An obvious rule applies to fading the signals in and out:

When splitting a signal into overlapping segments and recombining them, without changing the amplitudes in the frequency domain, the recombined signal must correspond exactly to the original signal.

In the time interval from 4 to 12 ms, all three segments contribute and the analog signal is complete. As soon as the procedure generates a fourth segment, the section 12 to 16 ms will also be complete.

Processing a continuous signal thus consists of the following five steps.

1. Split the continuous signal into successive, overlapping time segments

2. Fade the signal in at the start of each segment, and out again at the end

3. Transform each segment into the frequency domain, change the amplitudes in the spectrum by applying the desired multiplication factors, and transform each spectrum back into the time domain, as described in the previous section

4. Fade the signal in at the start of each segment and out again at the end

5. Add the overlapping segments to construct the continuous output signal

◆ Summary

In this chapter, we learned how to process a continuous signal with the Fourier transform. We first reviewed how the Fourier transform acts on simple sinusoidal signals. We also focused on processing a single segment, and extended the procedure to cope with continuous signals.

References

Beerends, R. J., ter Morsche, H. G., van den Berg, J. C., and van de Vrie, E. M. (2003). Fourier and laplace transforms. New York: Cambridge University Press.

Butz, T. (2005): Fourier transformation for pedestrians. New York/Heidelberg/Berlin: Springer.

Cooley, J. W., and Tukey, J. W. (1965). An algorithm for the machine computation of complex Fourier series. Mathematics of Computation, 19, 297–301.

Gauss, C.F. (1866). Nachlass: Theoria interpolationis methodo nova tractate, Königliche Gesellschaft der Wissenschaften, Göttingen, Germany. Werke Band, 3, 265–327.

Pappandreou-Suppappola, A. (2003). Applications in time-frequency signal processing. Boca Raton, FL: CRC Press.

Walker, J. S. (1996). Fast Fourier transforms (2nd ed.). Boca Raton, FL: CRC Press.

Zölzer U., Amatriain X., Arfib D., Evangelista G., Keiler F., Loscos A., Rocchesso D., Sandler M., Serra X., Todoroff T., Bonada J., De Poli G., and Dutilleux P. (2002). DAFX – Digital audio effects. Hoboken, NJ: John Wiley & Sons.

12

Digital Filters

This and the next two chapters differ from the previous ones. The focus is now on the calculations that take place in the hearing aid processor. This difference may require a different reading style, especially if a reader's domain excludes mathematical tasks.

The analysis here is not pure mathematics, however. The approach is to explain concepts by going through numerical examples. Nevertheless, just reading through the sections will hardly convey the knowledge. It may prove necessary to stop after each example, work through the calculations once more, and then perhaps read the text again.

This chapter is about a central topic in digital signal processing: filtering. You will see that digital signals are a series of numbers and that filtering consists of calculating with them. The sections in this chapter cover

1. *Digital test signals*: provides a few signals that the example filters will later work on

2. *Digital low- and high-pass filter*: introduces simple digital filters and makes it possible to grasp the idea behind digital signal processing (DSP) algorithms

3. *Wide dynamic range compression (WDRC) with a low- and high-pass filter*: uses the filters of the previous section and shows how to apply them in practice

4. *WDRC with a controllable finite impulse response (FIR) filter*: catches up on a topic from Chapter 5, the filter update mechanism of a controllable FIR filter

The analysis here uses Excel (Microsoft Corp., Redmond, WA) spreadsheets to demonstrate

calculations. This choice will allow most readers to retrace the examples. There are more suitable tools, however, MATLAB (MathWorks, Inc., Natick, MA), for example. Some textbooks present DSP theory alongside MATLAB examples: Ingle and Proakis (2006), Welch et al (2005), Kumar (2005), or Stearns (2002). Lyons (2004) is a best-selling, introductory textbook; Oppenheim et al (1999) and Rabiner and Schafer (1978) are classical references, and Proakis and Manolakis (2006) and Quatieri (2001) are two more widely used textbooks.

◆ Digital Test Signals

We first addressed digital signals in Chapter 5. The short overview introduced the notion of *sampling rate*: the number of samples per second taken from a continuous signal. For the sake of simplicity, the intention here is to derive signals that take only integer numbers; to this end the specification for the test signals is

◆ Sampling rate F = 6 kHz
◆ Cosine signals with
   Amplitude A = 16
   Frequencies f = 0, 1, 1.5, 2 and 3 kHz

The short overview of digital signals also mentioned typical sampling rates in hearing aids: 16 and 20 kHz. With these sampling rates the processing schemes provide for signals with a bandwidth of 8 and 10 kHz, respectively. In fact, this relation is the sampling theorem due to Claude Elwood Shannon, an American mathematician.

	A	B	C	D	E	F	G	H	I	J	K	L	M	N	O	P
1	Sampling rate [Hz]															
2	6000															
3	Sampling interval [s]															
4	0.000167															
5	Amplitude															
6	16															
7	pi															
8	3.14															
9	Time index	-2	-1	0	1	2	3	4	5	6	7	8	9	10	11	12
10	Frequency [Hz]															
11	0	0	0	16	16	16	16	16	16	16	16	16	16	16	16	16
12	1000	0	0	16	8	-8	-16	-8	8	16	8	-8	-16	-8	8	16
13	1500	0	0	16	0	-16	-0	16	0	-16	-0	16	0	-16	0	16
14	2000	0	0	16	-8	-8	16	-8	-8	16	-8	-8	16	-8	-8	16
15	3000	0	0	16	-16	16	-16	16	-16	16	-16	16	-16	16	-16	16

Figure 12–1   Calculation of the digital test signals.

A sampling rate of X kHz means that signal components with frequencies smaller than $^{1}/_{2} \cdot$ X kHz are allowed only.

The amount of $^{1}/_{2} \cdot$ X kHz is also known as the Nyquist frequency, named for the American physicist Harry Nyquist, who was born in Sweden and emigrated to the United States at the age of 18.

The frequency of 3 kHz for a cosine test signal in the specification above is no problem, however, although the sampling rate is just 6 kHz.

The Excel table in **Fig. 12–1** holds the samples of the test signals for time indices n = 0 to 12. Cells D11 to P11 show the samples of the first test signal, cells D12 to P12 those of the second test signal, cells D13 to P13 for the third test signal, and so on. All sample values are indeed integer numbers: 16, 8, 0, −8, and −16.

What does it take to generate the test signal samples? The list below holds step-by-step instructions, using Excel notation. If you need help understanding Excel notation, see Mac-Donald (2005).

1. Enter the sampling rate, F = 6 kHz, into cell A2: **6000**.

2. The duration T of a sampling interval is equal to $1/F$; so, in cell A4 enter the Excel formula: **=1/A2**.

3. For the amplitude of the waveform, A, enter the value **16** into cell A6.

4. In cell A8, store the value of π (pi). It would be possible to type in the rough value of 3.14; however, using the *arc tan* function delivers a value exact to many more decimal places: **=4*ATAN(1)**.

5. Enter the first time index n = −2 into cell B9. Signals usually start from time 0; here, however, it is necessary to prepare two earlier signal values for later use.

6. In cell C9, increase the time index n by 1: = **B9 + 1**.

7. Next drag (a spreadsheet action that designates *copying*) the formula from cell C9 to P9, thereby obtaining all time-indices up to 12.

8. Enter the test frequencies f into the cells A11 to A15: **0, 1000, 1500, 2000,** and **3000**.

9. In cells B11 to C15 arbitrarily set the sampled values of the test signals at times n = −2 and n = −1 to **0**.

10. Calculate the sample values of the test signals using the formula $A \cdot \cos(2 \cdot \pi \cdot f \cdot n \cdot T)$; into cell D11, enter the formula in Excel syntax: **=\$A\$6*COS(2*\$A\$8*\$A11*D\$9*\$A\$4)**.

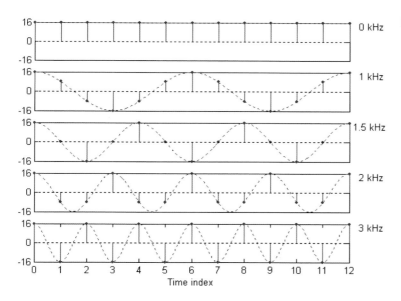

Figure 12–2   Digital test signals.

11. Next, drag the formula from cell D11 horizontally to cell P11, obtaining the sample values of the first test signal.

12. Drag cells D11 to P11 vertically down to row 15 to see the sample values of the four other test signals.

Figure 12–2 depicts the five test signals as a series of "pins" similar to the representation that was introduced in Chapter 5. The dotted curves show the continuous analog waveforms from which the digital samples are taken.

◆ Digital Low- and High-pass Filter

In this section, I will discuss two simple FIR filters. With a FIR filter, if the input signal to the filter has only one sample with a nonzero value, then the output signal will have only a finite number of nonzero samples. This is in contrast to IIR filters that we will review in the next chapter. IIR stands *for infinite impulse response*; an IIR filter's response to a singular nonzero input sample may take infinitely long to die away.

Digital filters are abstract constructions; they consist of a few numbers and a calculation procedure. Hence a mathematical formula is most suitable to describe a digital filter. The formula represents a filter in a compact form, but is not necessarily easy for everyone to understand.

It is also possible to represent the filters in a block diagram; although more intuitive, this approach still needs additional explanation.

As a result, the approach here is to

1. Describe our example of a FIR filter
2. Present a block diagram
3. Summarize the system using a mathematical formula

The Finite Impulse Response (FIR) Filter

Our examples of FIR filters rely on three numbers: their filter coefficients. Now, imagine the digital signal as a series of sample values that arrive one after the other at regular intervals. At any specific point calculate the sample value of the filtered output signal by performing the following four steps:

1. Multiply the current sample value by the first filter coefficient
2. Multiply the previous sample value by the second filter coefficient
3. Multiply the next previous sample value by the third filter coefficient
4. Sum the three products, to obtain the sampled value of the output signal

Then repeat the four-step procedure for each new input sample, and in this way calculate the complete filtered output signal.

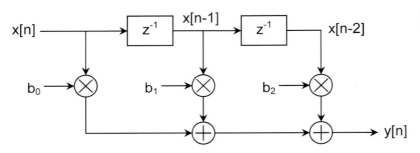

Figure 12–3   Digital finite impulse response filter.

The discussion so far has left a question open: what procedure provides suitable filter coefficients to achieve a desired transfer function? This topic, however, exceeds the scope of this book. For a discussion on filter design, see any of the DSP books referenced at the beginning of this chapter. The examples here use predefined filter coefficients.

Block Diagram

Figure 12–3 shows the block diagram of a simple FIR filter. The quantities $x[n]$ and $y[n]$ denote, respectively, the sampled input and output signals, at a specific point, n. The three filter coefficients are b_0, b_1, and b_2. In addition, the blocks marked z^{-1} delay the input signal by one sampling period; incidentally, z^{-1} is a typical notation in DSP systems.

The block diagram in **Fig. 12–3** contains three levels from top to bottom.

1. The top level provides the current sampled value of $x[n]$, and the previous sampled values of $x[n-1]$ and $x[n-2]$.

2. Arithmetic operators on the middle level multiply sample values of the input signal by the corresponding filter coefficients.

3. Arithmetic operators on the bottom level sum the products, giving the output signal $y[n]$.

Mathematical Formula

The symbols from the block diagram easily translate into the filter formula that is also referred to as a *difference equation*:

$$y[n] = b_0 \cdot x[n] + b_1 \cdot x[n-1] + b_2 \cdot x[n-2]$$
(Eq. 12-1)

This formula is a compact representation of both the block diagram and the text description. The next two subsections will apply the theory into practice.

Digital Low-pass Filter

Low- and high-pass filters follow the same calculation procedure. They only differ from one another in the choice of filter coefficients. For our low-pass filter, the coefficients are $b_0 = 1/4$, $b_1 = 1/2$, and $b_2 = 1/4$.

The Excel table in **Fig. 12–4** shows how the low-pass filter acts on the test signals from the first section. The test signal samples are again in cells D11 to P15, and the samples of the filtered signals are in cells D23 to P27.

What does it take to generate the Excel table? The process is as follows:

1. Enter the filter coefficients $1/4$, $1/2$, and $1/4$ in cells A18 to A20

2. Enter the filter formula $b_0 \cdot x[n] + b_1 \cdot x[n-1] + b_2 \cdot x[n-2]$ into cell D23 using the Excel syntax: = **\$A\$18*D11+\$A\$19*C11+\$A\$20*B11**

3. Drag this formula horizontally from D23 across to P23. This generates the output signal from filtering the first test signal.

4. Drag the formulae in cells D23 to P23 vertically downward to row 27. This generates the output signals obtained when filtering the four other test signals.

Figure 12–5 shows the waveforms of the filtered signals. The filter attenuates the test signals more and more as their frequency increases. Comparing the output signals with the input waveforms reveals an additional detail: the filter causes a delay of one sampling interval. In **Fig. 12–2**, the waveforms of the harmonic oscillations reach a peak value at $n = 6$, but the output signals in **Fig. 12–5** only reach the peak at time $n = 7$.

	A	B	C	D	E	F	G	H	I	J	K	L	M	N	O	P	Q
9	Time index	-2	-1	0	1	2	3	4	5	6	7	8	9	10	11	12	
10	Frequency [Hz]																
11	0	0	0	16	16	16	16	16	16	16	16	16	16	16	16	16	
12	1000	0	0	16	8	-8	-16	-8	8	16	8	-8	-16	-8	8	16	
13	1500	0	0	16	0	-16	-0	16	0	-16	-0	16	0	-16	0	16	
14	2000	0	0	16	-8	-8	16	-8	-8	16	-8	-8	16	-8	-8	16	
15	3000	0	0	16	-16	16	-16	16	-16	16	-16	16	-16	16	-16	16	
16																	
17	Low-pass filter																
18	1/4	b0															
19	1/2	b1															
20	1/4	b2															
21	Time index			0	1	2	3	4	5	6	7	8	9	10	11	12	
22	Frequency [Hz]																Gain
23	0			4	12	16	16	16	16	16	16	16	16	16	16	16	1
24	1000			4	10	6	-6	-12	-6	6	12	6	-6	-12	-6	6	3/4
25	1500			4	8	0	-8	0	8	0	-8	0	8	0	-8	0	1/2
26	2000			4	6	-2	-2	4	-2	-2	4	-2	-2	4	-2	-2	1/4
27	3000			4	4	0	0	0	0	0	0	0	0	0	0	0	0
28																	

Figure 12–4   Low-pass filtering.

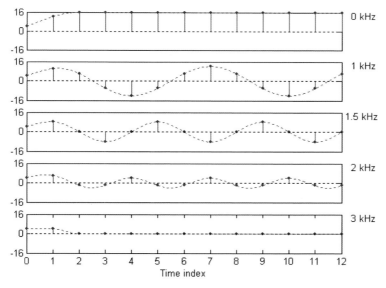

Figure 12–5   Output signals from the low-pass filter.

Let us quickly consider why this delay occurs. First, note that calculating an output sample involves the input samples from three subsequent time points. So, it is unrealistic to expect the output signal to have no delay at all. It seems rather natural that the output sample is valid for the middle of the time interval from which input samples contribute; and this thought leads to a delay of exactly one sampling period. This is no strict proof, of course; a derivation in the strict mathematical sense is, however, beyond the scope of this book. It is

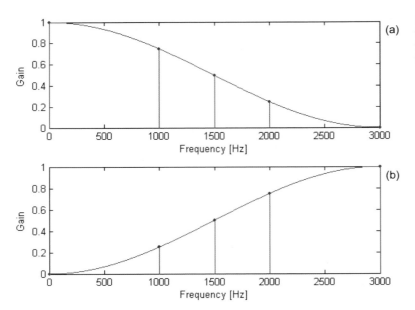

Figure 12–6 Transfer functions of **(a)** a FIR low-pass filter and **(b)** a FIR high-pass filter.

important to keep this filter delay in mind as the analysis proceeds to the next question: How much does the filter amplify the signal?

It is usual to talk of amplification, although the low-pass filter only passes a signal or attenuates it. To determine the amplification, divide the peak value of the output signal by the peak value of the input signal – continuing on from the previous steps:

5. Enter the formula **=K23/J11** into cell Q23: the low-pass filter amplifies the first test signal by 1.

6. Drag the formula from cell Q23 down to cell Q27; this yields the gain values for the remaining four test signals: $3/4$, $1/2$, $1/4$, and 0.

Figure 12–6a shows the transfer function of the low-pass filter. For the sake of simplicity, the diagram uses linear scales: neither logarithmic frequency nor logarithmic amplification in dB are used. The vertical lines in the diagram indicate the calculated gain values from the Excel table. They lie exactly on the continuous transfer function and thus confirm full agreement.

The low-pass filter lacks clear pass- and stop-bands. Significantly more than three filter coefficients would be needed to get a steep slope between pass- and stop-bands; or, in technical terms, a higher filter order would be needed.

Digital High-pass Filter

For a two-channel WDRC system it is desirable to have a high-pass filter with a transfer function that is complementary to that of the low-pass filter. The amplification of the two complementary filters should sum to 1 at every frequency.

Figure 12–6b shows the transfer function of this high-pass filter. Vertical lines at the frequencies 0, 1, 1.5, 2, and 3 kHz show by how much the high-pass filter should amplify the different test signals. The Excel table in **Fig. 12–7** reveals the suitable high-pass filter coefficients: $b_0 = -1/4$, $b_1 = 1/2$, and $b_2 = -1/4$.

The easiest way to get this table is to copy the previous example and change the filter coefficients b_0 and b_2 from $+1/4$ to $-1/4$. The formulae in the different cells then calculate the output signals and gains based on the high-pass filter coefficients.

Figure 12–8 shows the filtered signal waveforms. As the test signal frequency increases, the gain increases from 0 to 1. The result corresponds exactly to the expected transfer function shown in **Fig. 12–6b**.

	A	B	C	D	E	F	G	H	I	J	K	L	M	N	O	P	Q
9	Time index	-2	-1	0	1	2	3	4	5	6	7	8	9	10	11	12	
10	Frequency [Hz]																
11	0	0	0	16	16	16	16	16	16	16	16	16	16	16	16	16	
12	1000	0	0	16	8	-8	-16	-8	8	16	8	-8	-16	-8	8	16	
13	1500	0	0	16	0	-16	-0	16	0	-16	-0	16	0	-16	0	16	
14	2000	0	0	16	-8	-8	16	-8	-8	16	-8	-8	16	-8	-8	16	
15	3000	0	0	16	-16	16	-16	16	-16	16	-16	16	-16	16	-16	16	
16																	
17	High-pass filter																
18	- 1/4	b0															
19	1/2	b1															
20	- 1/4	b2															
21	Time index			0	1	2	3	4	5	6	7	8	9	10	11	12	
22	Frequency [Hz]																Gain
23	0			-4	4	0	0	0	0	0	0	0	0	0	0	0	0
24	1000			-4	6	2	-2	-4	-2	2	4	2	-2	-4	-2	2	1/4
25	1500			-4	8	0	-8	0	8	0	-8	0	8	0	-8	0	1/2
26	2000			-4	10	-6	-6	12	-6	-6	12	-6	-6	12	-6	-6	3/4
27	3000			-4	12	-16	16	-16	16	-16	16	-16	16	-16	16	-16	1
28																	

Figure 12–7 High-pass filtering.

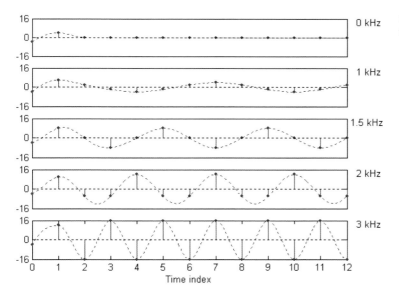

Figure 12–8 Output signals from the high-pass filter.

◆ Wide Dynamic Range Compression with a Low- and High-pass Filter

The digital low- and high-pass filters from the previous section make it possible to realize a

WDRC system. The analysis divides into the following four topics:

1. *Block diagram*: shows how the two filters fit into the picture
2. *All-pass characteristic*: explores how to accomplish a system that neither amplifies nor attenuates

3. *Time-invariant gain*: demonstrates how to establish a fixed gain curve

4. *Time-varying gain*: deals with changing the amplification over time, as usually occurs with WDRC

Block Diagram

In the block diagram of **Fig. 12–9,** the acoustic signal passes through a microphone and reaches an analog-to-digital converter. The output signal of the converter, x[n], feeds the inputs of the high- and low-pass filters. The next step involves multiplying the low-pass filter's output signal by a gain g_L and the high-pass filter's output signal by a gain g_H. The amplified band signals eventually reach an adder that fits the two signals together to form the output signal y[n]. The digital-to-analog (D/A) converter transforms y[n] into a continuous signal and forwards it to the receiver.

The block diagram in **Fig. 12–9** is a fragment; it excludes the blocks *level measurement* and *compression characteristic* that are part of a WDRC system. In this way, the block diagram holds for both processing schemes that were presented in Chapter 4, for two-channel WDRC and for two-band WDRC. In other words, a single broadband signal level may drive the compression characteristics – or two signal levels, one in the low and one in the high frequencies. Both options are valid.

All-pass Characteristic

With $g_L = 1$ and $g_H = 1$, the complementary characteristics of the two filters causes the output signal to be identical to the input signal, apart from a delay of one sampling period. This is easy to verify by adding together the filtered signal samples shown in **Fig. 12–4** and **Fig.**

12–7; the results are identical to the input signal samples in **Fig. 12–1**.

Time-invariant Gain

Now we turn to an example in which g_L and g_H have different values, thereby causing one frequency region to dominate. For instance, take the values $g_L = \frac{1}{2}$ and $g_H = 2$. These values cause the WDRC system to amplify the high-frequency signal components and attenuate the low frequencies. It is again possible to calculate the output signals by using the values from the tables in **Fig. 12–4** and **Fig. 12–7**.

The next step is to calculate the gain applied to each of the test signals as they pass through the block diagram. This is easy for the test signals with frequencies of 0 and 3 kHz. The 3 kHz test signal is exclusively in the upper band signal; the other is exclusively in the lower band signal. So, this yields an overall gain of 2 at 3 kHz and $\frac{1}{2}$ at 0 Hz.

The test signal with a frequency of 1.5 kHz is present in both bands at half its original amplitude. The two band signals thus evenly contribute, yielding an overall gain of $\frac{1}{2} \cdot \frac{1}{2} + 2 \cdot \frac{1}{2} = 1\frac{1}{4}$. Following the same reasoning for the other test signals yields the results as summarized in **Table 12–1**.

As an aside, the symbol g_{LP} in **Table 12–1** denotes how much the low-pass filter amplifies each test signal, and g_{HP} denotes how much gain the high-pass filter applies.

Figure 12–10 shows the transfer function. The gain from **Table 12–1** again agrees with the transfer function at the test frequencies of 0, 1, 1.5, 2, and 3 kHz.

Time-varying Gain

So far, the gains g_L and g_H were assumed to be constant. With the architecture in **Fig. 12–9** it

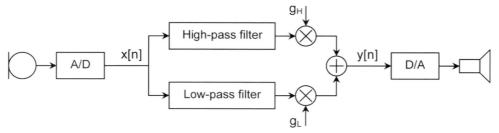

Figure 12–9 A two-channel wide dynamic range compression system.

Table 12–1   Calculation of Overall Gain for $g_L = \frac{1}{2}$ and $g_H = 2$

Frequency (Hz)	g_L		g_{LP}		g_H		g_{HP}		Overall Gain
0			1				0		1/2
1000			¾				¼		7/8
1500	½	×	½	+	2	×	½	=	1¼
2000			¼				¾		1 ⅝
3000			0				1		2

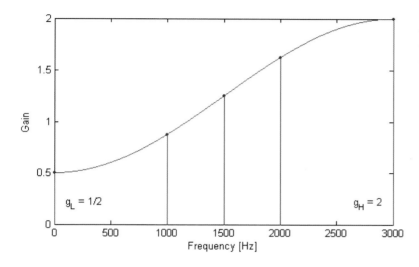

Figure 12–10   Transfer function of the two-channel wide dynamic range compression system, for $g_L = \frac{1}{2}$ and $g_H = 2$.

is, in fact, possible to vary them over time, from one sampling period to the next actually. In this way, the WDRC system can completely change its amplification every 50 μs – given that the sampling rate is 20 kHz, for example. This high rate of change looks a bit odd when put in contrast to commonly used WDRC time constant of 20 ms to 20 s, corresponding to a ratio of 1 : 400 to 1 : 400,000, respectively. This mismatch actually forms the reason for the controllable FIR filter to get into the picture.

◆ **Wide Dynamic Range Compression with a Controllable FIR Filter**

This section shows how to combine the separate low- and high-pass filters into a single controllable FIR filter. This approach will provide a

deeper understanding of the WDRC technique that we first looked at in Chapter 5.

The analysis here proceeds along the same four topics as with the WDRC system in the previous section: block diagram, all-pass characteristic, time-invariant gain, and time-varying gain. It, however, adds a fifth topic to discuss—the use of realistic controllable filters in hearing aids.

Block Diagram

Figure 12–11 shows the block diagram of a WDRC system using a controllable FIR filter. A single filter calculates the output signal y[n] in this scheme. The single filter, however, additionally requires a filter control block.

In a previous section, we determined that the low- and high-pass filters share the same filter architecture, but use different filter coefficients. The filter architecture also extends to the controllable FIR filter.

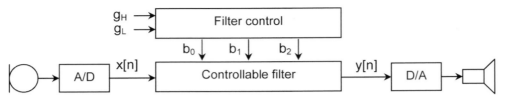

Figure 12–11   A wide dynamic range compression system using a controllable finite impulse response filter.

Table 12–2   Filter Coefficient Calculation for $g_L = 1$ and $g_H = 1$

	Low-pass Filter		High-pass Filter		Controllable Filter
b_0	¼		−¼		0
b_1	½	+	½	=	1
b_2	¼		−¼		0

All-pass Characteristic

To accomplish an all-pass characteristic, it is necessary to calculate the filter coefficients for $g_L = 1$ and $g_H = 1$. This requires adding together the low- and high-pass filter coefficients, as **Table 12–2** shows.

In the previous section, the WDRC system produced an output signal that was identical to the input signal, apart from a delay of one sampling period. It is easy to verify this fact; just enter the filter coefficients from **Table 12–2** into the filter formula:

$$y[n] = b_0 \cdot x[n] + b_1 \cdot x[n-1] + b_2 \cdot x[n-2]$$
$$= 0 \cdot x[n] + 1 \cdot x[n-1] + 0 \cdot x[n-2]$$
$$= x[n-1]$$

$$\text{(Eq. 12-2)}$$

That is at any time point n, the output sample $y[n]$ equals the input sample $x[n-1]$, where $n-1$ denotes the time point one sampling period before.

Time-invariant Gain

We will again look at the values $g_L = ½$ and $g_H = 2$. How is it possible to derive the suitable filter coefficients for the controllable filter? First, multiply the low-pass filter coefficients by g_L and the high-pass filter coefficients by g_H, then add the results together. **Table 12–3** illustrates the procedure.

Next, let us apply the filter coefficients in **Table 12–3** in another spreadsheet calculation. The easiest way to do this is to make a copy of one of the previous examples and enter the new filter coefficients:

$$b_0 = -3/8, \quad b_1 = 1¼, \quad \text{and} \quad b_2 = -3/8.$$

Figure 12–12 shows the resulting Excel table. Cells D23 to P27 contain the sample values of the output signals, and cells Q23 to Q27 show the gain values. These gain values agree with those in **Table 12–1**, and thus confirm the controllable filter to be equivalent to the two-channel WDRC system in the previous section.

Figure 12–13 shows the output signal waveforms. Because the maximum gain is 2, in this case, the y-axis has the range −32 to +32.

Time-varying Gain

As we have seen in the previous section, it is possible for the two-channel WDRC system to change the gain values g_L and g_H at every sampling interval. As noted there, this high rate of change looks a bit odd when compared with the time constants that WDRC systems commonly use. So, what factors determine a relevant time frame?

In Chapter 6, we ascertained how to measure the sound pressure level of an acoustic signal. As we saw there, the observation window defines the time segment from which sample values contribute to the measurement. The analysis showed that the level value has to stay constant for at least the duration of a phoneme, even when targeting a fast-acting WDRC system.

Now, recall the basic block diagram of a WDRC system from Chapter 4: the measured level value goes to a compression characteristic block that, in turn, defines how much to amplify the signal. The rate of change thus translates from the measured level to the desired gain. The

	A	B	C	D	E	F	G	H	I	J	K	L	M	N	O	P	Q
9	Time index	-2	-1	0	1	2	3	4	5	6	7	8	9	10	11	12	
10	Frequency [Hz]																
11	0	0	0	16	16	16	16	16	16	16	16	16	16	16	16	16	
12	1000	0	0	16	8	-8	-16	-8	8	16	8	-8	-16	-8	8	16	
13	1500	0	0	16	0	-16	-0	16	0	-16	-0	16	0	-16	0	16	
14	2000	0	0	16	-8	-8	16	-8	-8	16	-8	-8	16	-8	-8	16	
15	3000	0	0	16	-16	16	-16	16	-16	16	-16	16	-16	16	-16	16	
16																	
17	Controllabe filter																
18	- 3/8	b0															
19	1 1/4	b1															
20	- 3/8	b2															
21	Time index			0	1	2	3	4	5	6	7	8	9	10	11	12	
22	Frequency [Hz]																Gain
23	0			-6	14	8	8	8	8	8	8	8	8	8	8	8	1/2
24	1000			-6	17	7	-7	-14	-7	7	14	7	-7	-14	-7	7	7/8
25	1500			-6	20	0	-20	0	20	0	-20	0	20	0	-20	0	1 1/4
26	2000			-6	23	-13	-13	26	-13	-13	26	-13	-13	26	-13	-13	1 5/8
27	3000			-6	26	-32	32	-32	32	-32	32	-32	32	-32	32	-32	2

Figure 12–12   Processing with a controllable finite impulse response filter.

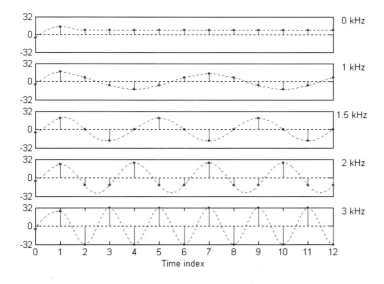

Figure 12–13   Output signals of a two-channel wide dynamic range compression system.

time constants in the measurement process usually range from around 10 ms to several seconds. Given a sampling rate of 20 kHz, for example, it is possible to completely update the filter during each sampling period (i.e., every 50 μs) but it would be overkill. Such frequent updates are not only unnecessary, but also cause excessive drain on battery power.

So, what is a suitable update mechanism for the controllable FIR filter? First, recall from **Table 12–3** how the filter coefficients of the low- and high-pass filters combine to form the filter coefficients b_0, b_1, and b_2 of the controllable filter. Let b_0^{LP}, b_1^{LP}, and b_2^{LP} denote the low-pass filter coefficients, b_0^{HP}, b_1^{HP}, and b_2^{HP} the coefficients of the high-pass filter, g_L the

Table 12–3   Filter Coefficient Calculation for $g_L = \frac{1}{2}$ and $g_H = 2$

	g_L		Low-pass Filter		g_H		High-pass Filter		Controllable Filter
b_0			¼				−¼		−³⁄₈
b_1	½	×	½	+	2	×	½	=	1 ¼
b_2			¼				−¼		−³⁄₈

gain for the low frequencies and g_H the gain for the high frequencies. Then:

$$b_0 = g_L \cdot b_0{}^{LP} + g_H \cdot b_0{}^{HP}$$
$$b_1 = g_L \cdot b_1{}^{LP} + g_H \cdot b_1{}^{HP}$$
$$b_2 = g_L \cdot b_2{}^{LP} + g_H \cdot b_2{}^{HP} \quad \text{(Eq. 12-3)}$$

The main idea of the new update mechanism is quite simple: from one sampling period to the next, update the controllable filter with respect to only one of its partial filters – for example, from time index $n - 1$ to time index n with respect to the low-pass filter:

$$b_0[n] = b_0[n - 1] - g_L[n - 2] \cdot b_0{}^{LP}$$
$$+ g_L[n] \cdot b_0{}^{LP} \quad \text{(Eq. 12-4)}$$

and similar equations for b_1 and b_2.

The equation means that you get the current value $b_0[n]$ by

1. Starting from the previous value $b_0[n - 1]$
2. Subtracting the last contribution of the low-pass filter from two sampling periods ago: $g_L[n - 2] \cdot b_0{}^{LP}$
3. Instead adding the currently required contribution: $g_L[n] \cdot b_0{}^{LP}$

It is possible to simplify the equation by rearranging the terms:

$$b_0[n] = b_0[n - 1] + (g_L[n] - g_L[n - 2]) \cdot b_0{}^{LP}$$
$$\text{(Eq. 12-5)}$$

In the next sampling period, it will be necessary to update the controllable filter with respect to the high-pass filter:

$$b_0[n + 1] = b_0[n] + (g_H[n + 1]$$
$$- g_H[n - 1]) \cdot b_0{}^{HP}$$
$$\text{(Eq. 12–6)}$$

and similar equations for b_1 and b_2.

The update procedure refreshes each constituent of the controllable filter every 100 µs – still sufficiently fast compared with typical time constants in WDRC systems. Although the update mechanism may seem to be of minor importance, it easily extends to multiple frequency bands and then proves to be very valuable.

Controllable Filters in Hearing Aids

A controllable FIR filter in a hearing aid must be made up of many band-pass filters to achieve a good target match; we looked at such an example once again in Chapter 5. Let us assume 20 partial filters to come close to the number of third-octave bands in the frequency range up to 10 kHz.

To obtain reasonably overlapping pass-bands, each band-pass filter needs ~100 filter coefficients. Calculating the output signal of a single filter represents a considerable effort in itself. Performing the calculations for 20 of these filters in parallel is completely impractical. In a hearing aid it is mandatory to save calculations and thereby keep power consumption within limits. At this point the controllable filter comes in handy, as does the fast Fourier transform (FFT) approach; however, the calculation details of the FFT are beyond the scope of this book.

The value of the controllable FIR filter is rooted in the update mechanism that we just reviewed, and in the fact that it easily extends to a filter with many constituent frequency bands. An example will make this clear: assume a sampling rate of 20 kHz and a controllable FIR filter being composed of 20 partial filters. This specification produces the following two key results.

1. The filter update mechanism completely refreshes the filter once per ms, namely, still

sufficiently often compared with the time constants that WDRC systems commonly use.

2. The computational burden boils down to roughly one tenth of a system that runs 20 fixed band-pass filters in parallel.

These two features make the controllable FIR filter an attractive option for implementing a WDRC system.

◆ Summary

In this chapter, we first learned how to calculate simple digital test signals. Then we explored digital low- and high-pass filters and their effect on the previously established test signals. We also saw how the digital filters were used in a WDRC system, first in a typical two-channel setup, and then as constituents of a controllable FIR filter.

The final topic focused on what it means to use a realistic controllable FIR filter in a hearing aid. The key to success is rooted in a suitable update mechanism that refreshes the filter sufficiently often to ensure high sound quality, and at the same time keeps the computational burden within limits, resulting in acceptable power consumption.

References

Ingle, V.K., and Proakis, J.G. (2006). Digital signal processing using MATLAB (2nd ed.). Toronto, Ontario, Canada: Thomson-Engineering.

Kumar, B.P. (2005). Digital signal processing laboratory. Boca Raton, FL: CRC Press.

Lyons, R.G. (2004). Understanding digital signal processing (2nd ed.). Englewood Cliffs, NJ: Prentice Hall.

MacDonald, M. (2004). Excel: The missing manual. Sebastopol, CA: O'Reilly Media.

Oppenheim, A.V., Schafer R.W., and Buck J.R. (1999). Discrete-time signal processing. Englewood Cliffs, NJ: Prentice Hall.

Proakis, J.G., and Manolakis, D.G. (2006). Digital signal processing (4th ed.). Englewood Cliffs, NJ: Prentice Hall.

Quatieri, T.F. (2001). Discrete-time speech signal processing: Principles and practice. Englewood Cliffs, NJ: Prentice Hall.

Rabiner, L.R., and Schafer, R.W. (1978). Digital processing of speech signals. Englewood Cliffs, NJ: Prentice Hall.

Stearns, S.D. (2002). Digital signal processing with examples in MATLAB. Boca Raton, FL: CRC Press.

Welch T.B., Wright C.H.G., and Morrow M.G. (2005). Real-time digital signal processing from MATLAB to C with the TMS320C6x DSK. Boca Raton FL: CRC Press.

13

Digital Level Measurement

In this chapter, we will determine how a digital hearing aid processes a signal to find its sound pressure level. An international standard (International Electrotechnical Commission [IEC], 2002) gives specifications for sound measuring instruments; it defines 125 ms as a fast time constant. In case of a burst noise, hearing instruments have to reduce the amplification much faster to avoid emitting too loud a sound; they thus have to depart from the standard when it comes to time constants. The sections in this chapter cover

1. *Overview of the measurement process*: discusses the processing steps to acquire the sound pressure level, including the averaging process that a low-pass filter usually performs

2. *Digital infinite impulse response (IIR) filter*: presents the averaging means that produces the decaying observation window discussed in Chapter 6

3. *Peak value and instantaneous value measurement*: describes variants of the IIR filter that make it possible to measure the sound pressure level as a peak value or as an instantaneous value, as outlined in Chapter 6

As stated in the previous chapter, the analysis here presents the calculations made by the digital hearing aid processor. Therefore, take your time and work through the details of the numerical examples. This should make the ideas clearer and the text easier to understand.

◆ **Overview of the Measurement Process**

The standard (IEC, 2002) describes the measurement process as a three-step procedure.

1. Square the input signal
2. Filter the squared signal with a simple low-pass filter
3. Map the filter's output signal onto a logarithmic scale

Without an expertise in measurement processes, these instructions may be puzzling; understanding the reasoning behind these steps should aid in the comprehension of the process.

What should a sound pressure level tell us? It should indicate the average sound pressure over a short period, and it should do so in a suitable format. Now, think of the sound pressure oscillations. They feature positive and negative half waves; averaging is thus likely to produce a value equal or close to zero, regardless of how big or small their amplitudes. In such a case, measurement processes often resort to a different average: the root-mean-square (RMS) value. The first instruction – squaring the input signal – indeed originates from the objective to calculate an RMS value.

As to the suitable format, Chapter 1 already addressed this issue. Sound pressure varies over an enormous range, and the sound pressure level represents this range on a manageable dB scale. Recall the relation between sound pressure and sound pressure level

$$L = 10 \cdot \log_{10}(p^2/p_0^2) = 20 \cdot \log_{10}(p/p_0)$$
$$\text{with } p_0 = 20 \ \mu\text{Pa.} \qquad \text{(Eq. 13-1)}$$

The third instruction – mapping onto a logarithmic scale – actually serves the purpose of expressing the measurement values in a handy dB format.

So far, one question remains: Why filter the squared input signal? The three-step RMS calculation provides a hint.

1. Square the signal
2. Take the average of the squared values
3. Evaluate the square root of the average

In fact, filtering aims at averaging the squared input signal. However, the term *averaging* generally associates with a seemingly different concept: given N numbers in a finite set, add them up and divide the sum by N. This kind of averaging also applies to calculating the sound pressure level when an algorithm processes the signal in segments, as with the transformation into the frequency domain described in Chapter 5, for example.

Most processing algorithms, however, update all quantities from sampling period to sampling period – for example, those using a filter bank and those using controllable filters as presented in Chapter 5. These processing algorithms require a running average, and here filtering comes in handy. There is a straightforward connection between filtering and the seemingly different averaging concept. Recall our discussion of the FIR filters in Chapter 12. For a moment,

assume a signal segment to consist of only three samples and set all three filter coefficients to one-third each. This FIR filter generates a running average following the familiar averaging concept.

Now, there remain some practical items to consider. To begin, you can easily extend the FIR filter to cope with larger segments. At a 20 kHz sampling rate, for example, a 10-ms signal segment holds 200 samples. An FIR filter with 200 filter coefficients would provide the running average in this case; each filter coefficient is set to 0.005. But two disadvantages make this approach impractical. First, the computational burden increases too much; and second, the average would lag the signal by 5 ms, that is, by half the segment length – similar to the one-sample delay that the three-tap FIR filter discussed in Chapter 12 exhibits.

Luckily, both issues vanish by using another filter type: the IIR filter, which we will examine in an upcoming section. With the IIR filter structure, generating the running average requires only one single filter coefficient. Also, the delay decreases dramatically, as a result of the decaying observation window that the IIR filter produces. Recall from Chapter 6 that this kind of observation window weights the recent signal sample more and previous samples less, the farther back in time they lie.

Let us now focus on the mainstream variants; **Fig. 13–1** shows their block diagrams. The first block in **Fig. 13–1a** is labeled *rectify*, a leftover of analog technology. It has found its way into some digital hearing aids, mainly because rectifying consumes less battery power than squaring.

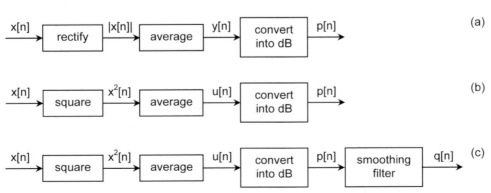

Figure 13–1   Block diagrams of the level measurement process: **(a)** with rectifying the input signal, **(b)** with squaring the input signal, and **(c)** with squaring the input signal and additional smoothing filter.

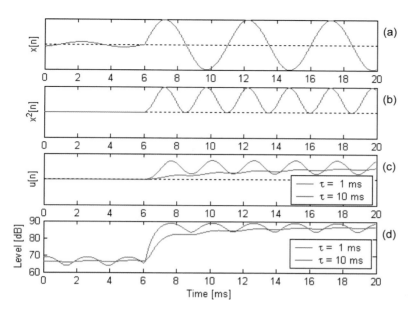

Figure 13–2 Signals produced by a level measurement: **(a)** sinusoidal test signal, **(b)** squared signal, **(c)** averaged squared signal, and **(d)** sound pressure level.

Figures 13–1b and **13–1c** both include *squaring* as a first step and thus comply with the international standard (IEC, 2002). All three block diagrams also comply with the standard regarding the second and third step: averaging and converting the average into dB. **Figure 13–1c** features an additional fourth step: a smoothing filter to postprocess the measurement value obtained in the first three steps. The smoothing filter is not part of the standard, but deals with the time constant issue.

Next, we will look at how the first, second, and third measurement step act on the test signal in **Fig. 13–2a**, a harmonic oscillation with a frequency of 200 Hz. Moreover, the test signal features a sound pressure level that jumps from 67 to 87 dB at time point 6 ms.

Squaring the Input Signal

Figure 13–2b shows the result of squaring the sinusoidal input signal: another harmonic oscillation with twice the frequency, and an offset such that all signal values are greater than or equal to zero. You may think of squaring as a means to turn negative signal values into positive ones, but there is more to it. If there was not, you might as well rectify the signal to get all signal values nonnegative. Nonetheless, rectifying only works in an approximate way; the mathematical details are beyond the scope of this book, however.

As a matter of fact, rectifying produces a measurement error that varies with the specific waveform that different signals exhibit; hence a fixed correction will only remove the error in the average. By contrast, the RMS approach produces accurate level values for all signal waveforms. The digital processor in a hearing instrument can simply and precisely square the input samples, unlike analog electronics that deals with the continuous input signal. Hence the RMS measurement should eventually end up in all digital hearing instruments.

However, squaring in the first step also has a slight drawback; it produces larger numerical values for the averaging process to deal with. We will address this issue below, presenting an IIR filter structure that is particularly suitable for this purpose.

Averaging

As outlined before, the averaging process consists in low-pass filtering. There is still a design option: How to set the bandwidth of the passband—or equivalently how to set its time constant. We will also look more closely at this relation in a later section.

Depending on the chosen value for the time constant, the filter will react more or less quickly when its input signal changes. **Figure 13–2c** shows the resulting average for two different time constants; a value of 1 ms causes the output signal to rise steeply and then show an output ripple synchronized to the squared signal. On the other hand, a time constant of 10 ms has the effect of slowing the initial rise, but produces a more stable output.

Converting to a dB Scale

Figure 13–2d shows the signal level after the digital processor has converted the average squared signal into dB. These levels behave in the same way as the average values at the output of the low-pass filter:

◆ With a time constant of $\tau = 1$ ms, the measured value rises quickly, but exhibits a considerable ripple.

◆ A time constant of $\tau = 10$ ms produces a stable measurement value, but only with a delay of around 10 ms.

Let us now look at how a hearing aid processor calculates the sound pressure level according to Equation 13–1. Evaluating the logarithm of a variable is not quite a straightforward task for a hearing aid processor, because it lacks a button labeled *LOG* – unlike any pocket calculator.

Mathematics, of course, provides methods such as power series; for more details, see Godement (2002). But the power series for the logarithm converges slowly and the approach altogether requires too much calculating. Luckily, it is possible to use a simple *look-up table* – a method that is widely used in numerical computing, see Frerking (1994).

Figure 13–3 illustrates Equation 13–1, showing sound pressure level versus the ratio of squared sound pressures p^2/p_0^2. Recall that $p_0 = 20$ μPa is the reference sound pressure; the diagram, therefore, shows 0 dB SPL for = $p^2/p_0^2 = 1$. In this diagram, the sound pressure level appears as a straight line because the x-axis uses a logarithmic scale. Let us see what interesting items the diagram further holds:

◆ In Chapter 1, a basic relationship was stated between sound pressure and sound pressure level: when the sound pressure doubles, the level increases by 6 dB. In this case the squared ratio quadruples and the diagram thus shows 6 dB SPL for $p^2/p_0^2 = 4$. Similarly, if the sound pressure doubles again (i.e., if $p/p_0 = 4$), then the squared ratio is already 16, and the diagram actually shows 12 dB SPL for $p^2/p_0^2 = 16$. As a consequence, when p^2/p_0^2 doubles, the sound pressure level increases by 3 dB only.

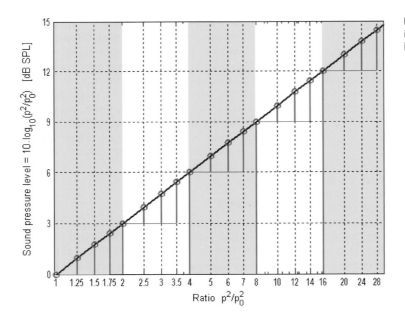

Figure 13–3   Principle of calculating sound pressure level using a look-up table.

◆ Due to the logarithmic scale, the distance between the values 1 and 2 on the x-axis is the same as the distance between the values 2 and 4, 4 and 8, and 8 and 16. This is similar to what we have already seen in Chapter 1: frequencies one octave apart from each other display at regular intervals on the logarithmic frequency-axis of a spectrum. This property also holds for proportions other than 1:2. For example, the distance between 1 and 1.25 is the same as between 2 and 2.5, 4 and 5, 8 and 10, and between 16 and 20. As a result of the straight line, the sound pressure level increases by the same amount when the ratio increases from 1 to 1.25, as when it increases from 2 to 2.5, 4 to 5, 8 to 10, or from 16 to 20. Given the level values of 3, 6, 9, and 12 dB SPL for the ratios of 2, 4, 8, and 16, respectively, it is just necessary to know the increase for a proportion of 1.25, to determine the sound pressure levels for the ratios of 2.5, 5, 10, and 20. This is also true for the proportions of 1.5 and 1.75 to determine the sound pressure levels for the ratios of 3, 3.5, 6, 7, 12, 14, 24, and 28.

What the analysis has revealed so far boils down to the mathematical law,

$$\log(c \cdot x) = \log(c) + \log(x) \qquad \text{(Eq. 13-2)}$$

that is, the logarithm of a product equals the sum of the logarithms of each factor.

Let us now see how the look-up table procedure works. **Table 13–1** shows how to calculate the sound pressure level for the squared sound pressures from 1,600 to 11,200 μPa^2, that is, for values of p^2/p_0^2 between 4 and 28. The fourth column in Table 13–1 holds the ratio values in a binary number representation in a computer or processor (Dandamudi, 2003; Dueck, 2004). To understand binary numbers, it is important to know the value that each digit has due to its position. Unlike the values 1, 10, 100, etc., in the decimal number system, the values are 1, 2, 4, etc., in the binary number system. Thus, for example,

$$111_{binary} = 1 \cdot 4 + 1 \cdot 2 + 1 \cdot 1 = 7 \text{ or}$$
$$10100_{binary} = 1 \cdot 16 + 0 \cdot 8$$
$$+ 1 \cdot 4 + 0 \cdot 2 + 0 \cdot 1 = 20.$$

The analysis above used the proportions 1:1.25, 1:1.5, and 1:1.75. There is a good reason to choose the values a quarter apart from each other; the binary numbers in **Table 13–1** reflect this choice in the two bits following the leading 1. Looking carefully at the table reveals how the table look-up procedure works; given a binary number for the ratio p^2/p_0^2, follow this two-step procedure to determine the sound pressure level.

Table 13–1   Calculation of Sound Pressure Level Using a Look-up Table

Squared Sound Pressure p^2 (μPa^2)	Ratio p^2/p_0^2 Decimal			Sound Pressure Level $10 \cdot \log_{10}(p^2/p_0^2)$ (dB SPL)
		Factors	Binary	
1,600	4	**4** · 1.00	**1**00	**6.0** + 0.0	6.0
2,000	5	**4** · **1.25**	**1**01	6.0 + **1.0**	7.0
2,400	6	**4** · **1.50**	**1**10	6.0 + **1.8**	7.8
2,800	7	**4** · **1.75**	**1**11	6.0 + **2.4**	8.4
3,200	8	**8** · 1.00	**1**000	**9.0** + 0.0	9.0
4,000	10	**8** · **1.25**	**1**010	9.0 + **1.0**	10.0
4,800	12	**8** · **1.50**	**1**100	9.0 + **1.8**	10.8
5,600	14	**8** · **1.75**	**1**110	9.0 + **2.4**	11.4
6,400	16	**16** · 1.00	**1**0000	**12.0** + 0.0	12.0
8,000	20	**16** · **1.25**	**1**0100	12.0 + **1.0**	13.0
9,600	24	**16** · **1.50**	**1**1000	12.0 + **1.8**	13.8
11,200	28	**16** · **1.75**	**1**1100	12.0 + **2.4**	14.4

The bold digits in the binary code correspond to the decimal factors and determine both a base value and an increment for the sound pressure level.

1. Determine the number N of bits following the leading 1 and multiply N by 3 dB to get a base value.
2. To the base value add an increment according to the two-bit pattern following the leading 1: 0 dB for pattern "00," 1 dB for "01," 1.8 dB for "10," and 2.4 dB for "11," respectively.

As outlined here, the procedure has a drawback: the sound pressure level increases in coarse steps of 1, 0.8, or 0.6 dB, respectively. It is easy, however, to extend the concept in practice. Instead of quarters, use eighth, sixteenth parts, or an even finer grid. As a result, the bit-pattern to consider grows to 3, 4, or more bits. Yet the complexity remains modest compared with evaluating the logarithm numerically.

◆ Digital Infinite Impulse Response Filter

In the previous chapter, digital FIR filters were presented and how to use them was illustrated in simple WDRC applications. The averaging task in level measurement provides a good opportunity to introduce another type of digital filter: the IIR filter. As already mentioned in previous chapters, the acronym IIR stands for *infinite impulse response*, that is, a singular nonzero input sample may cause the filter to produce an output signal that takes infinitely long to die away – at least in theory.

Our example of an IIR filter is particularly suitable to the averaging task because of its low computational burden: a single filter coefficient is sufficient to provide for a narrow pass-band and to effectively attenuate signal components at high frequencies. Often, however, IIR and FIR filters are suitable for a given task in practice.

How do the two filter types differ from one another? The FIR filter uses only input samples to calculate an output sample, whereas an IIR filter uses both the input samples and previously calculated output samples.

This section deals with three topics.

1. *Filter structure*: presents the block diagram of the simplest IIR filter and derives a variant that is suitable to cope with large numerical values
2. *Numerical example*: shows in detail how the arithmetic works
3. *Transfer function*: reveals how much the example filter attenuates signal components at different frequencies

Filter Structure

Figure 13–4a shows a block diagram of the simplest IIR filter that proves useful in many industrial applications; see Sinclair (2000) or Padmanabhan (2000).

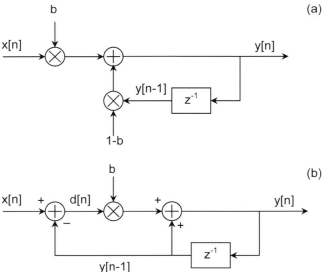

(a)

(b)

Figure 13–4   Digital IIR filter: **(a)** basic block diagram and **(b)** variant for dealing with large numeric values.

Figure 13–4b shows a variant of the schematic in **Fig. 13–4a**. This variant is particularly suitable for processing the larger values that the RMS measurement produces by squaring the input signal in the first processing step.

In the block diagrams,

◆ $x[n]$ and $y[n]$ represent, respectively, the input and output signal samples at time n

◆ The block marked z^{-1} represents a delay element, which provides

◆ $y[n-1]$, the previous output signal sample, at its output

◆ b and $(1-b)$ represent two filter coefficients

Filter coefficient b takes a value between 0 and 1, which makes the coefficient $(1-b)$ also lie within this range.

The block diagram in **Fig. 13–4a** shows how to calculate an output signal sample $y[n]$.

1. Multiply the current input sample $x[n]$ by filter coefficient b

2. Multiply the preceding output sample $y[n-1]$ by $(1-b)$

3. Sum the two products

This procedure is summarized in the formula,

$$y[n] = b \cdot x[n] + (1-b) \cdot y[n-1] \quad \text{(Eq. 13-3)}$$

What happens when the coefficient b takes different values? There are three cases.

1. $b = 0$: the filter formula becomes $y[n] = y[n-1]$, that is, the value of the output signal remains unchanged.

2. $b = 1$: the filter formula becomes $y[n] = x[n]$, that is, the input signal passes through unchanged.

3. $0 < b < 1$: a choice lying between the extremes produces an average of the input signal. This is different to the more common way of averaging in fixed segments. In that case, all sample values in the segment contribute equally to the average value; and those averages are calculated at regular intervals on consecutive, and sometimes overlapping, segments.

The IIR filter delivers a running average. At each sampling period, it weights the current input sample by the coefficient b, the average determined in the previous sampling period by $(1-b)$, and sums the two contributions.

The greater you choose b, the more the current input sample contributes to the average, the smaller is $(1-b)$ and the more quickly the influence of previous input samples decays. On the other hand, the smaller you choose b, the less the current input sample contributes to the average, the greater is $(1-b)$ and the less quickly the influence of previous input samples decays. This mechanism actually produces the decaying observation window that we defined in Chapter 6.

Next, it is possible to rearrange the filter formula and obtain a simpler form,

$$y[n] = b \cdot x[n] + (1-b) \cdot y[n-1] = b \cdot x[n]$$
$$+ y[n-1] - b \cdot y[n-1] = y[n-1]$$
$$+ b \cdot (x[n] - y[n-1]) \quad \text{(Eq. 13-4)}$$

The rearranged equation reflects the filter structure of the block diagram in **Fig. 13–4b**. The new filter structure saves a multiplication step compared with the previous diagram. In a next step, it is possible to further reduce the computational burden by choosing suitable values for the filter coefficient b, for example $b = 1/2$, $b = 1/4$, $b = 1/8$, etc. Just as multiplying a decimal number by 0.1, 0.01, or 0.001 is implemented by shifting the decimal point, multiplication by these values can be implemented by shifting the digits of a number represented in binary. This is especially beneficial when averaging the large numbers generated by the RMS measurement.

Here is how to calculate an output sample value $y[n]$, using the filter structure in **Fig. 13–4b**.

1. Subtract the previous output sample $y[n-1]$ from the current input sample $x[n]$ to get the difference $d[n]$

2. Multiply the difference $d[n]$ by the filter coefficient b

3. Add the product to the previous output sample $y[n-1]$

A numerical example will further elucidate the arithmetic process.

Numerical Example

We will look at how the low-pass filter reacts when its input signal suddenly changes, as in the example in the first section where the sound pressure level of a harmonic oscillation

	A	B	C	D	E	F	G	H	I	J	K	L
1	Time index	0	1	2	3	4	5	6	7	8	9	10
2	Test signal	0	0	512	512	512	512	512	512	512	512	512
3	Filter coefficient											
4	1/2	0	0	256	384	448	480	496	504	508	510	511
5	1/8	0	0	64	120	169	212	249	282	311	336	358
6	1/32	0	0	16	32	47	61	75	89	102	115	127
7	1/128	0	0	4	8	12	16	20	24	27	31	35

Figure 13–5   Calculation of the infinite impulse response filter-step response.

jumped from 67 to 87 dB SPL. For the sake of simplicity, the input signal in this example is less complex: it is 0 at the beginning and then jumps to the value 512 at a certain point. **Figure 13–5** shows an extract from an Excel table. It contains

◆ A time index with values from 0 to 10, in row 1

◆ A test signal with sample values stepping up from 0 to 512, in row 2

◆ Output signals from the IIR filter with filter coefficient values of $^1/_2$, $^1/_8$, $^1/_{32}$ and $^1/_{128}$ in rows 4 to 7, respectively

An example calculation using b = $^1/_2$ shows how the filter works:

$$y[1] = 0 + ^1/_2 \cdot (0 - 0) = 0 + 0 = 0$$
$$y[2] = 0 + ^1/_2 \cdot (512 - 0) = 0 + 256 = 256$$
$$y[3] = 256 + ^1/_2 \cdot (512 - 256)$$
$$= 256 + 128 = 384$$
$$y[4] = 384 + ^1/_2 \cdot (512 - 384)$$
$$= 384 + 64 = 448$$
$$y[5] = 448 + ^1/_2 \cdot (512 - 448)$$
$$= 448 + 32 = 480$$
$$y[6] = 480 + ^1/_2 \cdot (512 - 480)$$
$$= 480 + 16 = 496 \quad \text{etc.}$$

From time index $n = 2$ onward, the difference to the input signal always reduces by half.

To create the Excel table in **Fig. 13–5,**

1. Enter the time index values **0** to **10** in cells B1 to L1

2. In row 2, enter the test signal sample values: **0** in cells B2 and C2, **512** in cells D2 to L2

3. Enter the filter coefficients in cells A4 to A7: $^1/_2$, $^1/_8$, $^1/_{32}$, and $^1/_{128}$

4. Enter the starting output signal value of **0** in cells B4 to B7

5. In cell C4, enter the filter formula $y[n] = y[n-1] + b \cdot (x[n] - y[n-1])$ in Excel format: **=B4 + $A4*(C$2-B4)**

6. Drag (a spreadsheet action that designates *copying*) cell C4 horizontally across to cell L4; this generates the output signal for a filter coefficient $b = ^1/_2$

7. Drag cells C4 to L4 vertically down to row 7, generating the output signals for the remaining filter coefficients

Figure 13–6 displays the waveforms of the IIR filter's output signals. Comparing these signals to each other makes it clear: the smaller the value for filter coefficient b, the longer it takes the output signal to react to a step in the input signal.

Transfer Function

Now we turn our attention to the frequency domain. **Figure 13–7** shows the transfer function of the IIR filter for different values of filter coefficient b in a hearing aid working at a sampling rate of 20 kHz.

In electrical engineering, it is common to define the pass-band of a low-pass filter by the cutoff frequency, namely the frequency where the transfer function is at -3 dB relative to the pass-band. A difference of 3 dB refers to doubling a ratio of squared quantities, as the ratio p^2/p_0^2 in the previous section; and -3dB refers to halving a ratio of squared quantities. In connection with filters, the squared quantities refer to signal power. Assume a sinusoid with a frequency in the pass-band; the low-pass filter passes all its power. If its frequency equals the

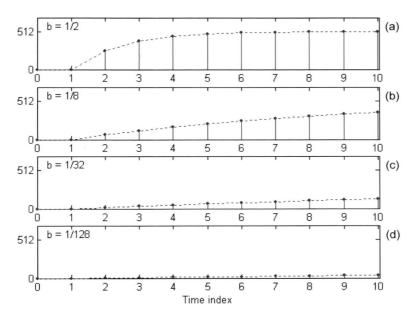

Figure 13–6   Waveforms of the infinite impulse response filter – step response for selected values of filter coefficient b: **(a)** b = ½, **(b)** b = ⅛, **(c)** b = 1/32, and **(d)** b = 1/128.

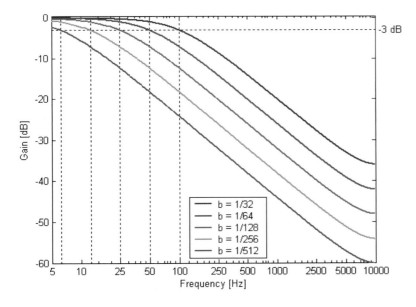

Figure 13–7   Infinite impulse response filter – transfer function for selected values of filter coefficient b.

cutoff frequency, however, then the low-pass filter passes only half of the signal power. The amplitude of the sinusoid is reduced by $\sqrt{1/2}$ in this case, by 0.707.

Table 13–2 summarizes values of the filter coefficient alongside cutoff frequencies and time constants, for the curves in **Fig. 13–7**. The table confirms the previous conclusion: the smaller the filter coefficient b, the nar-

rower the pass-band and the larger the time constant.

Measuring a sound pressure level with the low-pass filter described so far presents a problem that already became apparent in Chapter 6: the measurement process needs a short time constant to follow the short-time sound pressure level of consecutive phonemes. But then the periodic stimulus signal in voiced sounds

Table 13–2 Pass-band and Time Constants for Selected Values of Filter Coefficient b, Assuming a Sampling Rate of 20 kHz

Filter-coefficient b	Cutoff Frequency (Hz)	Time Constants (ms)
1/32	100	1.6
1/64	50	3.2
1/128	25	6.4
1/256	12	12.8
1/512	6	25.6

carries through to the measured value, and via the compression characteristic to the amount of amplification that a WDRC system applies, finally resulting in sound degradation. The analysis in Chapter 6 outlined two methods to cope with the problem: measuring a *peak value* or an *instantaneous value*. Both approaches slightly alter the structure on an IIR low-pass filter, as will be revealed in the next section.

◆ Peak Value and Instantaneous Value Measurement

In this section, the numerical details of the *peak value* measurement and the *instantaneous value*

measurement, as outlined in Chapter 6 are presented. Both approaches start from the filter structure in **Fig. 13–4b** and vary the filter coefficient b depending on the difference sample d[n].

1. *Peak value measurement*: uses two different values for the filter coefficient b, depending on the sign of the sample d[n]

2. *Instantaneous value measurement*: varies the filter coefficient b in the smoothing filter, depending on the magnitude of the sample d[n]

Peak Value Measurement

The peak value measurement is based on using two values for filter coefficient b: one if the difference d[n] is bigger than or equal to zero, the other if it is less than zero. It is always greater than zero when the sound pressure level is increasing, and smaller than zero when it is decreasing. This follows the principle, described in Chapter 6, of using different time constants for increasing and decreasing sound pressure levels.

To understand the process better, we turn to **Fig. 13–8**. It shows the output of the low-pass filter when the input signal steps back down from 512 to 0. The output signal goes down just as fast or slowly as it went up in the previous case, when the input signal stepped up to 512 – depending on the choice of filter coefficient b.

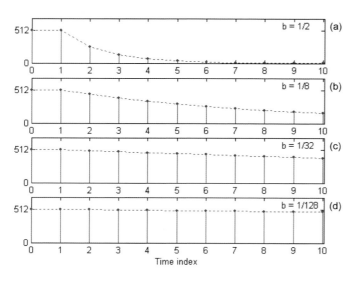

Figure 13–8 Waveforms of infinite impulse response filter-output signal when the input signal steps back down to zero, for selected values of filter coefficient b: **(a)** b = ½, **(b)** b = ⅛, **(c)** b = ¹⁄₃₂, and **(d)** b = ¹⁄₁₂₈.

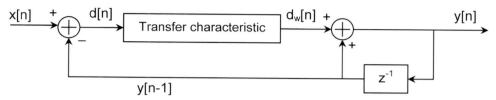

Figure 13–9 Smoothing filter as a low-pass infinite impulse response filter with a nonlinear transfer characteristic.

Using different values of b allows us to create a filter with asymmetric time constants. For instance, the values used in **Fig. 13–6a** and in **Fig. 13–8d** produce an extreme example.

◆ $b = 1/2$ for rising sound levels; then the average value at the output reaches the maximum input level after only a few sampling intervals

◆ $b = 1/128$ for falling sound levels; then the average value remains near to the previous maximum for a few hundred sampling intervals

For a signal such as speech, where the sound level constantly fluctuates between large and small values, such filter coefficient values cause the measurement to rapidly reach a peak and then remain more or less static. We have already seen this effect when measuring the sound pressure level of a speech signal in Chapter 6. The measured value in fact exceeds the true sound pressure level. The discussion there postponed the explanation why the effect occurs; now it is time to catch up.

Low-pass filtering serves the purpose of averaging the squared sound pressure samples. Using only one-time constant results in weighting positive and negative difference samples $d[n]$ equally; small and large squared signal samples then contribute to the same extent, thus yielding the true mean value. Using two different time constants, however, creates different weights for positive and negative difference samples $d[n]$. As a result, large squared sample values contribute more than small ones and the output signal rises above the true mean value.

Instantaneous Value Measurement

In the first section, we looked at an overview of level measurement and the block diagram

in **Figure 13–1c** introduced a *smoothing filter* (Schaub & Leber, 2002) to postprocess a raw value of the sound pressure level. As with the peak measurement, the *smoothing filter* again processes the difference value $d[n]$ differently, but this time based on the magnitude of $d[n]$ rather than its sign. For small difference values $d[n]$, the filter sets the coefficient b to be very small, and for large values it makes b much larger. Therefore, the output signal reacts sluggishly to small fluctuations in the input signal, but swiftly follows a large jump.

Figure 13–9 shows the block diagram of the *smoothing filter*. Instead of multiplying the difference $d[n]$ by filter coefficient b, there is now a block entitled *transfer characteristic*. We see in **Fig. 13–10** what this transfer characteristic looks like. The vertical axis shows the weighted level difference $d_w[n]$ passed on to the adder, for an input difference value $d[n]$ shown on the horizontal axis. For a standard IIR filter, b is fixed and the weighted difference $d_w[n]$ is always a fixed fraction of $d[n]$; for example, if $b = 1/2$, $d_w[n]$ is half of $d[n]$. This relationship appears in **Fig. 13–10** as a series of straight lines, with slopes depending on the value of b.

On the other hand, the bold purple line shows the *nonlinear transfer characteristic* that a typical *smoothing filter* implements. As a consequence, the filter

◆ Nearly blocks difference values $d[n]$ between -5 dB and $+5$ dB

◆ Increasingly passes difference values $d[n]$ that are less than -5 dB or greater than $+5$ dB

◆ Completely passes difference values $d[n]$ that are less than -12 dB or greater than $+12$ dB, i.e., $d_w[n] = d[n]$ in this case

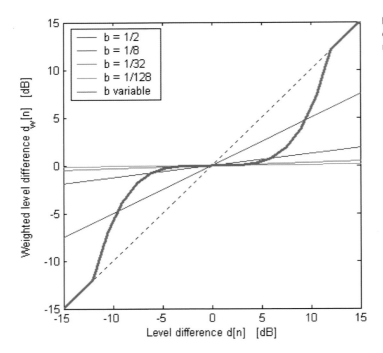

Figure 13–10 Transfer characteristics of a smoothing filter, and standard infinite impulse response filters.

◆ Summary

In this chapter we looked at the sequence of processing steps that a digital hearing aid uses to determine the sound pressure level of an acoustic signal: squaring the input signal, establishing a running average, and finally converting this average into a dB level.

The second processing step—averaging— involves an IIR filter. We reviewed the basic filter structure, as well as three variations: one for dealing with large numerical values, one for measuring a peak value, and one for measuring an instantaneous value.

References

Dandamudi, S.P. (2003). Fundamentals of computer organization and design. New York/Heidelberg/Berlin: Springer.

Dueck, R.K. (2004). Digital design with CPLD applications and VHDL. Clifton Park, NY: Thomson Delmar Learning.

Frerking, M.E. (1994). Digital signal processing in communications system. New York/Heidelberg/Berlin: Springer.

Godement, R. (2002). Analysis I: Convergence, elementary functions. New York/Heidelberg/Berlin: Springer.

International Electrotechnical Commission. (2002). IEC 61672-1. Electroacoustics – Sound level meters. Part 1: Specifications. Geneva, Switzerland: International Electrotechnical Commission.

Padmanabhan, T.R. (2002). Industrial instrumentation: Principles and design. New York/Heidelberg/Berlin: Springer.

Schaub, A., and Leber, R. (2002). Loudness-controlled processing of acoustic signals. United States Patent, US 6,370,255 B1, Apr. 9.

Sinclair, I.R. (2000). Audio and Hi-Fi handbook (3rd ed.). Woburn MA: Newnes.

14

Autocorrelation and Prediction

In this chapter, I will present the mathematical background of sound classification. As Chapter 10 outlined, sound classification aims at distinguishing different signals from one another, starting from suitable signal attributes such as sound pressure level, modulation, periodicity, spectral envelope parameters, etc. The sections in this chapter cover

1. *Autocorrelation*: shows how to calculate the autocorrelation coefficient and how the coefficient relates to periodicity

2. *Prediction*: presents the mathematical framework of spectral envelopes, prediction filters, and the normalized prediction error

This chapter is once more about mathematical concepts. The approach still consists in conveying knowledge by means of examples. Nevertheless, to grasp the ideas requires carefully studying the details step by step and sometimes rereading the text. For a thorough mathematical discussion of autocorrelation, see Chu (2003), Baken and Orlikoff (2000), or Goldberg and Riek (2000); with respect to prediction, refer to Greenberg et al (2004), Zölzer et al (2002), or Wade (1994).

If you lack expertise in mathematics, the terms *autocorrelation* and *prediction* may appear completely abstract to you. So, let us first consider the motivation for analyzing these issues.

Chapter 10 outlined the basics of signal classification. Extracting suitable attributes from the acoustic signal allows a hearing aid to classify the signal into one of several categories: speech, music, and monotonic or impulse noise. This, in turn, makes it possible to adjust the

mode of operation such that a hearing impaired listener benefits the most.

In the simplest case, this approach helps to overcome the shortcomings of a traditional noise reduction system that evaluates modulation only. As discussed in Chapter 3, such a noise reduction system fails in two typical situations: (1) with music and (2) with impulse noise, for example, when doing the dishes.

Music often features only little modulation; a noise reduction system then repeatedly attenuates the broadband signal or just some frequency bands, thus degrading the sound quality. Impulse noise, on the other hand, has considerable modulation. A noise reduction system hence fails to attenuate this kind of noise, although hearing-impaired listeners would appreciate if the hearing aid reduced the gain in this case as well.

Recall from Chapter 10 that both the periodicity and the spectral envelope help to distinguish signals from one another: music from monotonic noise and impulse noise from speech. The autocorrelation coefficient is the quantity that lets a hearing aid processor recognize whether a signal is periodic – and if so, what the period is. The diagrams in the Periodicity section in Chapter 10 depicted this characteristic, using a color code; in this chapter, I will show how to calculate it.

Furthermore, the normalized prediction error indicates to what degree it is possible to predict the short-term progress of a signal waveform. The diagrams in the Spectral Envelope section in Chapter 10 showed how this attribute varies for signals of different categories. The normalized prediction error thus

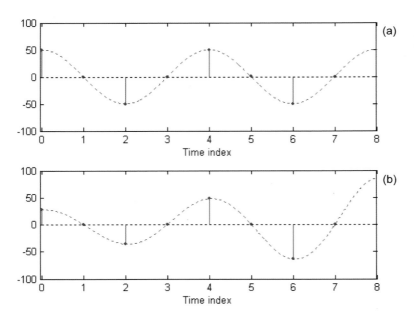

Figure 14–1   Test signals for calculating autocorrelation: **(a)** with constant amplitude and **(b)** with increasing amplitude.

also helps to classify signals. And in this chapter, I will show how to calculate it.

Note that prediction is different from periodicity. The time span of interest is shorter than the period of most signals, usually 1 ms or less. The examples in this book analyze how two or three subsequent signal samples depend on one another; assuming a sampling rate of 20 kHz, the time span is thus 100 μs, that is, just one tenth of a millisecond.

What happens in such a short time frames interrelates with the gross shape of a signal's spectrum. This is one of the interesting aspects reviewed in this chapter. Finally, grasping these concepts is likely to require a great deal of concentration simply because the topics exceed the basic level of signal processing theory.

◆ Autocorrelation

The term *autocorrelation* comes from Latin, and means *self-matching*. It concerns the relation between two segments of the same signal, more precisely, between the current segment and one that dates back a short period. To compare the two segments it is necessary that they have the same length. What segment length suits best depends on properties of the signal. If the frequencies of all signal components exceed a certain lower limit, then the inverse of this minimum frequency – the maximum period – is a suitable value for the segment length; and it is also a suitable value for the maximum time delay to consider between two segments. The minimum frequency of audio signals is around 50 Hz; hence 20 ms is a reasonable value for the segment length and also for the maximum time delay between two segments.

The analysis here starts from the two example signals that **Figs. 14–1a** and **14–1b** show. As usual, the dotted curves represent the continuous waveforms, and the "pins" mark the sample values at integer time points. Both diagrams illustrate two periods of a harmonic oscillation. In **Fig. 14–1a** the amplitude has a constant value of 50; in **Fig. 14–1b** the amplitude increases from 27 to over 80. The simpler case of a constant amplitude is the first example to investigate.

Test Signal with Constant Amplitude

The Excel table in **Fig. 14–2** shows how to calculate the autocorrelation coefficient for the test signal in **Fig. 14–1a**. Row 1 holds a time index n ranging from 0 to 7 and row 2 holds the signal samples $x[n]$: 50, 0, -50, 0, 50, etc.

	A	B	C	D	E	F	G	H	I
1	Time index n	0	1	2	3	4	5	6	7
2	Sample x[n]	50	0	-50	0	50	0	-50	0
3	Time delay k				4	3	2	1	0
4	Autocorrelation R(k)				5000	0	-5000	0	5000
5	Autocorrelation coefficient r(k)				1	0	-1	0	1

Figure 14–2   Calculation process for the autocorrelation coefficient of a test signal with constant amplitude.

First, it is necessary to define a segment length for the investigation. The test signal has a period that lasts four sampling intervals and this makes a suitable segment length in this example. A yellow background and a black border mark the current segment in the table: the samples $x[4]$ in cell F2, $x[5]$ in cell G2, $x[6]$ in cell H2, and $x[7]$ in cell I2. As a result, the samples $x[3]$ to $x[6]$ in cells E2 to H2 constitute a segment that dates back one sampling interval; the value 1 for the time delay k in cell H3 reflects this fact. Similarly, the samples $x[2]$ to $x[5]$ in cells D2 to G2 constitute a signal segment that dates back two sampling intervals, as the time delay $k = 2$ in cell G3 indicates. Then, the time delay $k = 3$ in cell F3 refers to the signal segment $x[1]$ to $x[4]$ in cells C2 to F2. And finally, the time delay $k = 4$ in cell E3 holds for the signal segment $x[0]$ to $x[3]$ in cells B2 to E2.

The next step consists of calculating the autocorrelation for each time delay value, from $k = 4$ to $k = 0$. According to the definition of autocorrelation, perform the following steps to obtain the result for the time delay $k = 4$, that is, the autocorrelation $R(4)$:

1. Multiply $x[0]$ by $x[4]$, yielding 2,500
2. Multiply $x[1]$ by $x[5]$, yielding 0
3. Multiply $x[2]$ by $x[6]$, yielding 2,500
4. Multiply $x[3]$ by $x[7]$, yielding 0
5. Sum up the four products, yielding $R(4) = 5,000$

The Excel table shows the autocorrelation $R(4)$ in cell E4, right below the time delay $k = 4$ in cell E3.

Next, to obtain the autocorrelation $R(3)$, multiply $x[1]$ by $x[4]$, $x[2]$ by $x[5]$, $x[3]$ by $x[6]$, $x[4]$ by $x[7]$, and sum up the four products. In each product one of the factors is zero; as a result,

the Excel table shows $R(3) = 0$ in cell F4. In the same way you obtain $R(2) = -5,000$ in cell G4, $R(1) = 0$ in cell H4, and $R(0) = 5,000$ in cell I4.

What has the analysis revealed so far?

◆ For a delay of a full period, the autocorrelation takes the maximum value – as in the case with no offset (i.e., $k = 0$), where the autocorrelation refers to only the current signal segment: $R(4) = R(0) = 5,000$.

◆ For a half period delay the signals are in antiphase and the autocorrelation takes the opposite value: $R(2) = -R(0) = -5,000$.

◆ For $k = 1$ and $k = 3$ the signals lie relative to one another such that one signal always has value 0 while the corresponding value from the other segment is $+50$ or -50. This results in $R(1) = 0$ and $R(3) = 0$.

If the amplitude of the test signal were not 50, but only 30 for example, then there would be a smaller maximum value: $R(4) = R(0) = 1800$. This indicates that the processor in the hearing aid should not take the autocorrelation value $R(k)$ directly, but should instead use a normalized value. Dividing $R(k)$ by $R(0)$ yields the normalized autocorrelation coefficient $r(k)$ in row 5. This normalization yields: $r(4) = r(0) = 1$, $r(2) = -1$ and $r(1) = r(3) = 0$; as intended, these values are independent of the signal amplitude.

The normalized autocorrelation coefficient $r(k)$ is a decisive factor for the processor to determine whether a signal is periodic. If it is, then, for a particular time delay k, $r(k)$ will take the value 1. Or it will at least approach the value 1 because the shape of a signal often alters naturally from one period to the next – due to a small noise signal, for example, that is superimposed on top of it.

The processor recognizes the period of the signal as being the smallest value k for which the autocorrelation coefficient $r(k)$ reaches its maximum. When the signal segments are delayed by integer multiples of a period, then the autocorrelation coefficient will again reach the maximum level.

The list below shows how to create the Excel table in **Fig. 14–2**. The instructions in this chapter use some advanced Excel syntax; if you need to consult a manual, see MacDonald (2005). To establish the table, proceed as follows:

1. Enter time index $n = \mathbf{0}$ into cell B1

2. In cell C1, enter the formula: = **B1+1**; this yields time index $n = 1$

3. Next, drag the formula from cell C1 to cell I1, obtaining all integer time indices up to $n = 7$

4. Fill the sample values from the test signal into cells B2 to I2: **50, 0, −50, 0, 50, 0, −50**, and **0**

5. Insert the time delay formula into cell E3: = **$I1-E1**; this produces $k = 4$

6. Drag the formula from cell E3 to cell I3, thereby obtaining the time delays down to $k = 0$

7. Enter the formula for $R(4)$ into cell E4: = **SUMPRODUCT(B2:E2,$F2:$I2)**. This gives $R(4) = 5000$

8. Drag the formula from cell E4 to cell I4, resulting in the values $R(3)$ to $R(0)$

9. Type the formula for the autocorrelation coefficient $r(4)$ into cell E5: = **E4/$I4**, producing $r(4) = 1$

10. Drag the formula from cell E5 to cell I5, generating the autocorrelation coefficients $r(3)$ to $r(0)$

The test signal with increasing amplitude in **Fig. 14–1b** slightly complicates the procedure. This is the next case we investigate.

Test Signal with Increasing Amplitude

The Excel table in **Fig. 14–3** shows how to calculate the autocorrelation coefficient for the test signal in **Fig. 14–1b**. Up to row 4, the procedure is identical to the previous example, except of course that row 2 contains different samples: 27, 0, −36, 0, 48, 0 −64, 0.

Normalizing the autocorrelation $R(k)$ to the autocorrelation coefficient $r(k)$ needs more care in this example. In general, dividing by the autocorrelation $R(0)$ produces an inaccurate result. The normalized coefficient $r(k)$ becomes slightly too small when the amplitude increases, and too large when the amplitude decreases – occasionally $r(k)$ gets even greater than 1.

How is it possible to obtain a meaningful value in all cases? To this end, it is necessary to first see where the problem originates. The autocorrelation $R(k)$ emanates from the samples in two signal segments, the current segment and the one that dates back k sampling intervals. The samples from only one segment, however, contribute to the normalization quantity $R(0)$; recall from the previous example that $R(0)$ equals the sum of squares of the samples in the current signal segment. Hence, to obtain a meaningful autocorrelation coefficient, replace the equation

$$r(k) = R(k)/R(0) \qquad \text{(Eq. 14-1)}$$

with

$$r(k) = R(k)/\sqrt{R(0)} \cdot \sqrt{SS(k)} \qquad \text{(Eq. 14-2)}$$

where $SS(k)$ denotes the sum of squares of the samples in the segment that dates back k sam-

	A	B	C	D	E	F	G	H	I
1	Time index n	0	1	2	3	4	5	6	7
2	Sample x[n]	27	0	-36	0	48	0	-64	0
3	Time delay k				4	3	2	1	0
4	Autocorrelation R(k)				3600	0	-4800	0	6400
5	SS(k)				2025	3600	3600	6400	6400
6	Root(SS(k))				45	60	60	80	80
7	Autocorrelation coefficient r(k)				1	0	-1	0	1
8									

Figure 14–3   Calculation process for the autocorrelation coefficient of a test signal with increasing amplitude.

pling intervals. For example, to obtain SS(4), perform the following steps.

1. Square the sample $x[0]$, yielding 729
2. Square the sample $x[1]$, yielding 0
3. Square the sample $x[2]$, yielding 1296
4. Square the sample $x[3]$, yielding 0
5. Sum up the four square values, yielding 2025

The Excel table shows the sum of squares SS(4) in cell E5. Next, to obtain SS(3), square $x[1]$, $x[2]$, $x[3]$, $x[4]$, and sum up the square values; the Excel table holds SS(3) = 3,600 in cell F5. In the same way you obtain SS(2) = 3,600 in cell G5, SS(1) = 6,400 in cell H5, and SS(0) = 6,400 in cell I5; SS(0) equals $R(0)$.

Row 6 holds the square roots of the sum of squares: $\sqrt{SS(4)}$ = 45 in cell E6, $\sqrt{SS(3)}$ = 60 in cell F6, $\sqrt{SS(2)}$ = 60 in cell G6, $\sqrt{SS(1)}$ = 80 in cell H6, and $\sqrt{SS(0)}$ = $\sqrt{R(0)}$ = 80 in cell I6.

Finally, row 7 shows the autocorrelation coefficients $r(k)$ = $R(k) / (\sqrt{SS(k)} \cdot \sqrt{SS(0)})$: $r(4)$ = 1 in cell E7, $r(3)$ = 0 in cell F7, $r(2)$ = −1 in cell G7, $r(1)$ = 0 in cell H7, and $r(0)$ = 1 in cell I7. The calculation procedure thus recognizes that the signal segments match, even if the amplitude monotonically increases, and would also do so if it were to monotonically decrease.

The list below holds the instructions to generate the Excel table. The first eight steps are the same as in the previous list; I therefore continue with step 9.

9. Enter the formula to calculate SS(4) into cell E5: **= SUMSQ(B2:E2)**; this produces the result 2025
10. Drag the formula from cell E5 to I5, generating the remaining normalizing quantities
11. In cell E6, type the square root formula: **= SQRT(E5)**, which gives the result 45
12. Drag the formula from cell E6 to I6, thereby obtaining the roots of the other normalizing quantities
13. Enter the formula for the autocorrelation coefficient $r(4)$: **= E4/(E6*$I6)**, resulting in $r(4)$ = 1
14. Drag the formula from cell E7 to cell I7, obtaining the remaining autocorrelation coefficients $r(3)$ to $r(0)$

The calculation examples have demonstrated the method that the processor in the hearing aid uses to calculate the autocorrelation coefficient.

◆ Prediction

This section will present the mathematical background of prediction and spectral envelopes, as outlined in Chapter 10. The gross shape of its spectrum reflects how well prediction works with a particular signal. It is possible to reasonably predict the waveform of a signal that has a spectrum with a steep gradient or with a pronounced resonance. On the other hand, any attempt will fail to predict the waveform of white noise; its spectrum is completely flat. In the Spectral Envelope Section in Chapter 10, the normalized prediction error was introduced to quantify how well prediction works. How all these quantities interrelate is the topic of this section; it divides into the following two subsections:

1. *Resonance filters*: will analyze two particular IIR filters, namely, filters with the same structure as the one used to establish a running average in Chapter 13. The analysis will show how their transfer functions depend on the values of their filter coefficients.

2. *Prediction filters*: will start from a new test signal with a flat spectrum; it will serve as the input signal to the resonance filters from the previous subsection. While processing the test signal, a resonance filter will imprint its transfer function on the test signal: the filtered test signal will thus feature a spectrum that is equal in shape to the transfer function of the filter.

In a next step, the analysis will show how to transform the resonance filters into prediction filters. The prediction filters will exhibit the inverse transfer function of the resonance filters. They will therefore again remove the spectral gradient and resonance from the spectrum of the filtered test signal and extract the predictable part from its waveform.

Finally, the analysis will show how to calculate the coefficients of a prediction filter and how to compute the normalized prediction error.

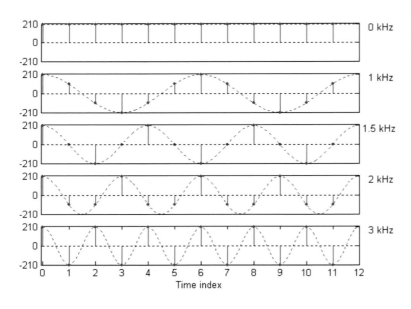

Figure 14–4   The waveforms of digital test signals for the resonance filters.

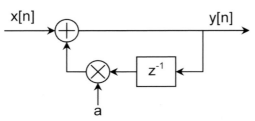

Figure 14–5   Block diagram of first-order resonance filter.

Resonance Filters

This subsection starts from the test signals reviewed in the first section in Chapter 12. The analysis here, however, requires increasing their amplitudes from 16 to 210, i.e., adjusting cell A6 in the Excel table of **Fig. 12–1**. This adjustment produces the test signals in **Fig. 14–4**. The larger amplitudes ensure that all numerical examples ahead will produce integer sample values, making the calculations simple to verify.

Next, we will look at two different resonance filters. **Figure 14–5** shows the block diagram of a first-order filter and **Fig. 14–6** of a second-order filter. Both block diagrams contain delay elements labeled "z^{-1}." These blocks are typical in signal processing schemes, as we have seen in Chapters 12 and 13. At its output, a delay element provides the sample value that was present at its input during the previous sampling period.

The first-order resonance filter generates an output sample $y[n]$ by

1. Multiplying the previous output sample $y[n-1]$ by the filter coefficient a
2. Adding the result to the current input sample $x[n]$

The filter formula thus is:

$$y[n] = x[n] + a \cdot y[n-1] \quad \text{(Eq. 14-3)}$$

The second-order resonance filter in **Fig. 14–6** produces an output sample $y[n]$ by

1. Multiplying the previous output sample $y[n-1]$ by the filter coefficient a_1
2. Multiplying the output sample $y[n-2]$ from two sampling intervals before by the filter coefficient a_2
3. Summing the two products together with the current input sample $x[n]$

The filter formula thus is:

$$y[n] = x[n] + a_1 \cdot y[n-1] + a_2 \cdot y[n-2] \quad \text{(Eq. 14-4)}$$

By examining the filter structures, it is clear that the second-order resonance filter incorporates the first-order filter within it. Setting $a_2 = 0$ and $a_1 = a$ yields identical filters.

Next, the analysis will apply the resonance filters to the test signals from **Fig. 14–4**. There are three cases to distinguish.

x[n]   y[n]

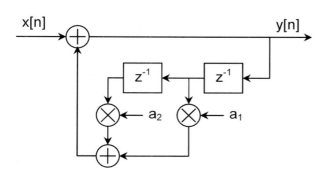

Figure 14–6 Block diagram of second-order resonance filter.

	A	B	C	D	E	F	G	H	I	J	K	L	M	N	O
9	Time index n	0	1	2	3	4	5	6	7	8	9	10	11	
10	Frequency [Hz]													
11	0	210	210	210	210	210	210	210	210	210	210	210	210	
12	1000	210	105	-105	-210	-105	105	210	105	-105	-210	-105	105	
13	1500	210	0	-210	-0	210	0	-210	-0	210	0	-210	0	
14	2000	210	-105	-105	210	-105	-105	210	-105	-105	210	-105	-105	
15	3000	210	-210	210	-210	210	-210	210	-210	210	-210	210	-210	
16														
17	Filter coefficient													
18	a	1/2												
19	Time index n	-1	0	1	2	3	4	5	6	7	8	9	10	11
20	Frequency [Hz]														Gain
21	0	420	420	420	420	420	420	420	420	420	420	420	420	420	2.00
22	1000	0	210	210	0	-210	-210	0	210	210	0	-210	-210	0	1.15
23	1500	-84	168	84	-168	-84	168	84	-168	-84	168	84	-168	-84	0.89
24	2000	-120	150	-30	-120	150	-30	-120	150	-30	-120	150	-30	-120	0.76
25	3000	-140	140	-140	140	-140	140	-140	140	-140	140	-140	140	-140	0.67
26														

Figure 14–7 Calculation process for a first-order resonance filter with filter coefficient $a = \frac{1}{2}$.

1. With positive coefficient a, the first-order filter amplifies the low frequencies, and attenuates the mid and high frequencies.

2. With negative coefficient a, the first-order filter amplifies the high frequencies, and attenuates the mid and low frequencies.

3. With the right choice of coefficients a_1 and a_2, the second-order filter amplifies the mid frequencies and attenuates the low and high frequencies.

First-Order Resonance Filter with Positive Filter Coefficients

The Excel table in **Fig. 14–7** illustrates the calculation procedure for the first-order reso-nance filter. Rows 11 to 15 show the sample values for the test signals from **Fig. 14–4**, and cell B18 contains the filter coefficient $a = \frac{1}{2}$.

Rows 21 to 25 show the sample values from the output signals. In contrast to previous examples, the assumption here is that the test signals have already driven the filter for negative time indices. In the Digital IIR Filter section of Chapter 13, we have seen that it takes the filter some time to react, when the samples at its input were constantly zero and then suddenly a nonzero signal appears. In the example here, however, the filter has already settled to steady-state; it therefore exhibits a starting value for time index n = −1 in column B, for example 420 in cell B21.

The next step in the analysis is to calculate the gain that the filter applies to each of the test signals. In Chapter 12, we learned how to proceed in the case of finite impulse response (FIR) filters. There, it was possible to calculate the ratio of amplitudes in the output and input signal, respectively. This was because those FIR filters delay all test signals by exactly one sampling period. Here, the situation is more complicated.

Figure 14–8 illustrates the waveforms of the filtered signals. Comparing these waveforms to the ones in **Fig. 14–4** reveals that the filter delays each test signal by a different period of time, by different fractions of a sampling interval actually. Hence the procedure here has to resort to calculating the ratio of RMS values. To obtain the gain values in cells O21 to O25, perform the following steps.

1. Square the output samples $y[n]$ and sum up the squared values

2. Take the square root of the sum

3. Square the input samples $x[n]$ and sum up the squared values

4. Take the square root of this second sum

5. Divide the first square root by the second

The gain values in the Excel table and the illustration in **Fig. 14–8** reflect the same finding: the filter amplifies the test signals in the low frequencies and attenuates those in the mid and high frequencies. After passing through the filter, the first test signal has the constant value 420: the filter amplifies it by a factor of 2. On the other hand, the 3 kHz signal in **Fig. 14–8** has an amplitude of 140, and the filter accordingly attenuates it by the factor $^2/_3$.

It is beyond the scope of this book to derive the gain for any frequency of test signal. **Figure 14–9a** shows the continuous transfer functions for the filter coefficient values $a = 0$, $a = {}^1/_4$, $a = {}^1/_2$, and $a = {}^3/_4$. The gain values from the Excel table are also marked onto **Fig. 14–9a**, as spot values of the red gain curve for $a = {}^1/_2$.

Comparing the different transfer functions in **Fig. 14–9a** reveals the following rule:

> The closer the filter coefficients are to 0, the flatter the transfer function – and on the other hand: the larger the chosen filter coefficients, the steeper the transfer function.

The list of instructions below demonstrates how to generate the Excel table in **Fig. 14–7**.

1. Enter the filter coefficient $a = {}^1/_2$ in cell B18

2. In cells B21 to B25 insert the initial values for time $n = -1$: **420, 0, −84, −120, −140**

3. Type the filter formula $x[n] + a \cdot y[n-1]$ into cell C21, using the Excel syntax: **= C11 + $B$18*B21**

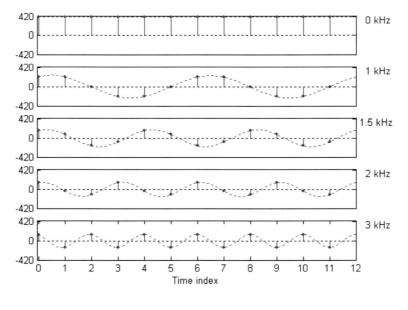

Figure 14–8   Waveforms of the output signals from the first order resonance filter with filter coefficient $a = {}^1/_2$.

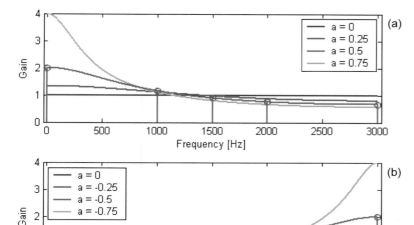

Figure 14–9 Transfer functions of the first-order resonance filter with different filter coefficient values: **(a)** positive coefficients and **(b)** negative coefficients.

4. Drag the filter formula horizontally from cell C21 to cell N21, generating the sample values from the output signal when the filter processes the first test signal

5. Drag the formula in cells C21 to N21 vertically down to row 25; this gives the sample values from the output signals, when the filter processes the remaining test signals

6. Enter the formula for calculating the gain into cell O21, using the Excel syntax: = **SQRT(SUMSQ(C21:N21))/SQRT(SUMSQ(C11: N11))**. This is the amount of gain the filter applies to the first test signal.

7. Drag the formula from cell O21 vertically down to cell O25, calculating the amount of amplification the filter applies to the other test signals

First-Order Resonance Filter with Negative Filter Coefficients

Figure 14–9b shows the transfer function of the first-order resonance filter for filter coefficients less than, or equal to 0. With negative filter coefficients, the transfer function increases as the frequency goes up – in contrast to the falling transfer function in **Fig. 14–9a**.

Comparing the different transfer functions in **Fig. 14–9b** shows how it is possible to generalize the rule from the previous section:

The larger the magnitude of the filter coefficient, the steeper is the transfer function.

The Excel table in **Fig. 14–10** contains the individual calculation steps for the example with a filter coefficient of $a = -\frac{1}{2}$. The easiest way to create this table is to copy the table from the previous example, change the filter coefficient in cell B18 to $-\frac{1}{2}$, and change the initial values in cells B21 to B25 to 140, 120, 84, 0, and -420.

The gain values in cells O21 to O25 also appear marked on the red transfer function in **Fig. 14–9b**, and confirm its rising gradient for the negative filter coefficient $a = -\frac{1}{2}$.

The output signal waveforms in **Fig. 14–11** again match the calculations in the Excel table. This time the filter amplifies the 3 kHz signal by a factor of 2, and attenuates the one with constant sample values by a factor of $\frac{2}{3}$.

Second-Order Resonance Filter

The Excel table in **Fig. 14–12** illustrates the calculation process for the case where a second-order resonance filter processes the test signals, using the filter coefficients $a_1 = 0$ and $a_2 = -\frac{1}{2}$.

Rows 11 to 15 again contain the various input signals, and cells B18 and B19 the two filter coefficients. As before, this table also calculates the output signals for the filter having settled to

	A	B	C	D	E	F	G	H	I	J	K	L	M	N	O
9	Time index n		0	1	2	3	4	5	6	7	8	9	10	11	
10	Frequency [Hz]														
11	0		210	210	210	210	210	210	210	210	210	210	210	210	
12	1000		210	105	-105	-210	-105	105	210	105	-105	-210	-105	105	
13	1500		210	0	-210	-0	210	0	-210	-0	210	0	-210	0	
14	2000		210	-105	-105	210	-105	-105	210	-105	-105	210	-105	-105	
15	3000		210	-210	210	-210	210	-210	210	-210	210	-210	210	-210	
16															
17	Filter coefficient														
18	a	- 1/2													
19	Time index n	-1	0	1	2	3	4	5	6	7	8	9	10	11	
20	Frequency [Hz]														Gain
21	0	140	140	140	140	140	140	140	140	140	140	140	140	140	0.67
22	1000	120	150	30	-120	-150	-30	120	150	30	-120	-150	-30	120	0.76
23	1500	84	168	-84	-168	84	168	-84	-168	84	168	-84	-168	84	0.89
24	2000	0	210	-210	0	210	-210	0	210	-210	0	210	-210	0	1.15
25	3000	-420	420	-420	420	-420	420	-420	420	-420	420	-420	420	-420	2.00
26															

Figure 14–10   Calculation process for a first-order resonance filter with filter coefficient $a = {}^{-}\tfrac{1}{2}$.

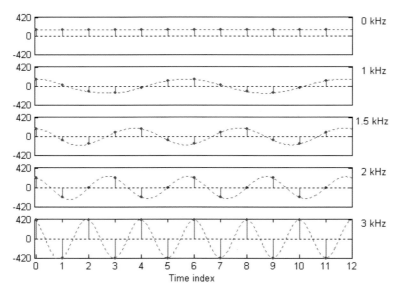

Figure 14–11   Waveforms of the output signals from the first-order resonance filter with filter coefficient $a = {}^{-}\tfrac{1}{2}$.

steady state; this time, however, two start values are necessary because the filter needs two earlier output samples. The Excel table holds them in cells B22 to B26 and C22 to C26.

Rows 22 to 26 show the output signals, and cells P22 to P26 the gain that the filter applies to the different test signals.

Figure 14–13 presents the output signal waveforms. The gain values in the Excel table and the waveforms in the illustration reflect the same finding: the filter amplifies the 1.5 kHz signal by a factor of 2, and attenuates the test signals with frequencies of 0 and 3 kHz by a factor of $^2/_3$.

	A	B	C	D	E	F	G	H	I	J	K	L	M	N	O	P
9	Time index n			0	1	2	3	4	5	6	7	8	9	10	11	
10	Frequency [Hz]															
11	0			210	210	210	210	210	210	210	210	210	210	210	210	
12	1000			210	105	-105	-210	-105	105	210	105	-105	-210	-105	105	
13	1500			210	0	-210	0	210	0	-210	0	210	0	-210	0	
14	2000			210	-105	-105	210	-105	-105	210	-105	-105	210	-105	-105	
15	3000			210	-210	210	-210	210	-210	210	-210	210	-210	210	-210	
16																
17	Filter coefficient															
18	a1	0														
19	a2	-1/2														
20	Time index n	-2	-1	0	1	2	3	4	5	6	7	8	9	10	11	
21	Frequency [Hz]															Gain
22	0	140	140	140	140	140	140	140	140	140	140	140	140	140	140	0.67
23	1000	0	210	210	0	-210	-210	0	210	210	0	-210	-210	0	210	1.15
24	1500	-420	0	420	0	-420	0	420	0	-420	0	420	0	-420	0	2.00
25	2000	0	-210	210	0	-210	210	0	-210	210	0	-210	210	0	-210	1.15
26	3000	140	-140	140	-140	140	-140	140	-140	140	-140	140	-140	140	-140	0.67

Figure 14–12   Calculation process for a second-order resonance filter with filter coefficients $a_1 = 0$ and $a_2 = -\frac{1}{2}$.

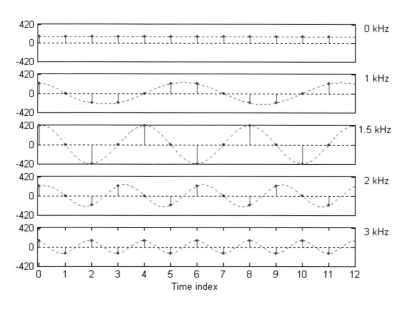

Figure 14–13   Waveforms of the output signals from the second-order resonance filter with filter coefficients $a_1 = 0$ and $a_2 = -\frac{1}{2}$.

Figure 14–14a shows the transfer function of the second-order resonance filter for different values of a_1, and a constant value $a_2 = -\frac{1}{2}$. The gain values from the Excel table are also marked as spot values for the transfer function for $a_1 = 0$ and $a_2 = -\frac{1}{2}$, given in red.

Comparing the various transfer functions in **Fig. 14–14a** reveals the rule:

Positive values of filter coefficient a_1 pull the resonance to lower frequencies, and negative values to higher frequencies. At the same time, the maximum gain increases.

Figure 14–14b shows the transfer functions for $a_1 = 0$ and various values of a_2, revealing the following rule:

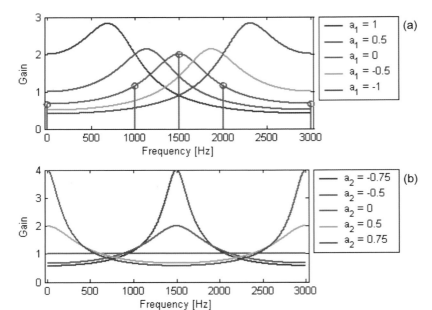

Figure 14–14 Transfer functions of the second-order resonance filter for different values of filter coefficients a_1 and a_2 **(a)** with $a_2 = {}^-\frac{1}{2}$ and **(b)** with $a_1 = 0$.

Negative values of filter coefficient a_2 produce a resonance – becoming stronger, with increasing magnitude; and positive values cause the filter to attenuate the mid frequencies, while at the same time amplifying both the low and high frequencies.

To conclude this example, here are the individual steps used to generate the Excel table in **Fig. 14–12**.

1. Enter filter coefficients $a_1 = $ **0** and $a_2 = {}^-\frac{1}{2}$ into cells B18 and B19

2. Put the initial values for time $n = -2$ into cells B22 to B26: **140, 0, −420, 0,** and **140**

3. Put the initial values for time $n = -1$ into cells C22 to C26: **140, 210, 0, −210,** and **−140**

4. Type the filter formula $x[n] + a_1 \cdot y[n - 1] + a_2 \cdot y[n-2]$ in cell D22, using the Excel syntax: **= D11+$B$18*C22+$B$19*B22**

5. Drag the formula from cell D22 horizontally to cell O22, generating the sample values of the output signal, created when the filter processes the first test signal

6. Drag cells D22 to O22 vertically down to row 26, to obtain the sample values of the output signals, created when the filter processes the remaining four test signals

7. Enter the formula to calculate the gain into cell P22, using the Excel syntax: **= SQRT(SUMSQ** **(D22:O22))/SQRT(SUMSQ(D11:O11))**. The filter amplifies the first test signal with the value 0.67.

8. Drag the formula from cell P22 vertically to cell P26. These are the gains that the filter applies to the other four test signals.

Prediction Filters

In Chapter 1, various noise signals were presented and it was noted that white noise has a flat spectrum. In reality, however, this only holds for the envelope of its spectrum, and the spectrum itself randomly oscillates around this envelope.

In fact, signals with precisely flat spectra do exist. They are of minimal practical use, however, as all but one of their samples have a value of zero. On the other hand, these signals are ideal for theoretical purposes, for instance, to illustrate prediction with simple example calculations.

This subsection is about prediction filters. Nevertheless, the analysis will take a short detour. To check how prediction filters work, it is desirable to provide suitable test signals with an exactly flat spectrum. Then, as the resonance filters from the previous subsection will filter a new test signal, the filtered output signal will exhibit a spectrum that is equal in shape to the transfer function of the resonance filter that produced it.

As we proceed to the numerical examples ahead, we will come across two surprises. Given the samples of an output signal, it is possible

1. To calculate the filter coefficients that were used in the resonance filter to generate them
2. To calculate the normalized prediction error, even without running a prediction filter

As seen in Chapter 10, one would usually run a prediction filter and calculate a difference signal to assess how well prediction works. Item 2 above states that these steps are altogether superfluous. The numerical examples ahead will actually use both approaches and demonstrate that they lead to identical results.

We will now turn to the detailed analysis of prediction filters. As with the resonance filters, there are also three cases to distinguish:

1. First-order prediction with positive filter coefficients
2. First-order prediction with negative filter coefficients
3. Second-order prediction

First-Order Prediction with Positive Filter Coefficients

Figure 14–15 shows the Excel table for the first example calculation. The time index n is given in the first row, and the new test signal $u[n]$ in the second. At time $n = 0$ it has the value 512,

and is otherwise 0. Cell B4 holds the filter coefficient $a = \frac{1}{2}$.

With the input signal $u[n]$ the resonance filter generates the output signal $x[n]$ in row 5.

Cells M6 and M7 contain the autocorrelation values $R(0)$ and $R(1)$ of the signal $x[n]$. They allow us to determine the coefficient that the resonance filter used while generating the signal $x[n]$ – as seen from cell M8 that contains the ratio $R(1) / R(0) = \frac{1}{2}$.

Next, let us see how to achieve prediction, starting from the resonance filter in **Fig. 14–5**. This takes the following thee steps.

1. Reverse the side branch that contains the delay element and the multiplier
2. Interchange the branching point and the adder
3. Replace addition by subtraction

Performing these steps yields the block diagram in **Fig. 14–16**. The part with yellow background represents the prediction filter, as introduced in Chapter 10. To obtain a sample $d[n]$ of the difference signal,

1. Multiply the previous input sample $x[n - 1]$ by the filter coefficient a, thus generating the estimate $y[n]$
2. Subtract the estimate $y[n]$ from the current input sample $x[n]$

In the Excel table, the first-order prediction generates the difference signal $d[n]$ in row 10 from the signal $x[n]$ in row 5. The difference

	A	B	C	D	E	F	G	H	I	J	K	L	M
1	Time index n	-1	0	1	2	3	4	5	6	7	8	9	
2	u[n]	0	512	0	0	0	0	0	0	0	0	0	
3	Filter coefficient												
4	a	1/2											
5	x[n]	0	512	256	128	64	32	16	8	4	2	1	
6	R(0)												349525
7	R(1)												174762
8	R(1) / R(0)												0.50
9	Prediction filter												
10	d[n]		512	0	0	0	0	0	0	0	0	0	
11	Normalized prediction error												0.75
12	k1 = R(1) / R(0)												0.50
13	V = 1 - k1*k1												0.75

Figure 14–15 Calculation process for first-order prediction with filter coefficient $a = \frac{1}{2}$.

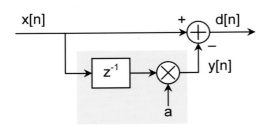

Figure 14–16   Block diagram of first-order prediction.

signal $d[n]$ precisely matches the test signal $u[n]$ in row 2, so prediction works in exactly the opposite way to the resonance filter.

As noted before, there are two ways to calculate the normalized prediction error. The first approach consists in calculating a ratio of sums of square values, following these three steps:

1. Square the difference samples $d[n]$ and sum up the squared values

2. Square the input samples $x[n]$ and sum up the squared values

3. Divide the first sum by the second

In our example, this procedure yields the value $3/4$ in cell M11.

Rows 12 and 13 present the alternative approach. First, it is necessary to calculate a new quantity, called the reflection coefficient:

$$k_1 = R(1)/R(0) \qquad \text{(Eq. 14-5)}$$

Cell M12 holds this value. For the first-order filter the reflection coefficient is equal to filter coefficient a.

Reflection coefficients are used in filters featuring a different structure to the one shown in **Fig. 14–16**. The topic is beyond the scope of this book; however, for a thorough discussion, see Zaknich (2005), Padmanabhan et al (2003), or Vaton et al (2002). The analysis here simply shows how to calculate the normalized prediction error V in cell M13, starting from the new quantity k_1:

$$V = 1 - (k_1)^2 \qquad \text{(Eq. 14-6)}$$

In our example, the calculation yields: $V = 1 - (1/2)^2 = 1 - 1/4 = 3/4$. Therefore, the values in cells M13 and M11 match precisely. In other words, the two ways of calculating the normalized prediction error agree exactly.

Figure 14–17a shows the waveforms of the signals from our example: The signal $x[n]$ is shown in blue, and the sample value $d[0]$ in green. **Figure 14–17b** shows their spectra. The spectrum of the signal $x[n]$ is shown in blue; it decreases with increasing frequency; the peak in the low-frequency range means that the waveform $x[n]$ decays monotonically, that is, without oscillation. On the other hand, the spectrum of the singular pulse signal $d[n]$ is completely flat. As prediction removes the predictable part of the signal $x[n]$, it flattens its spectrum at the same time.

The following list summarizes how to generate the Excel table in **Fig. 14–15**.

1. Enter time index **−1** into cell B1

2. Type the formula for this value plus one, into cell C1: **= B1 + 1**

3. Drag the formula from cell C1 to cell L1. This provides the time indices up to $n = 9$.

4. Enter the signal values $u[n]$ into cells B2 to L2: **512** in cell C2, **0** everywhere else

5. Put the filter coefficient value $1/2$ in cell B4

6. Type the initial value of **0** for time $n = -1$ into cell B5

7. In cell C5, program the filter formula $u[n] + a \cdot x[n - 1]$ using the Excel syntax: **= C2 + $B4*B5**, resulting in $x[0] = 512$

8. Drag the formula from cell C5 to cell L5, producing the remaining sample values for the signal $x[n]$

9. Enter the formula for the autocorrelation value $R(0)$ into cell M6, using the Excel syntax: **= SUMSQ(C5:L5)**. This gives $R(0) = 349,525$.

10. Enter the formula for the autocorrelation value $R(1)$ into cell M7, using the Excel syntax: **= SUMPRODUCT(C5:L5,B5:K5)**. This gives $R(1) = 174,762$.

11. Put the formula for the quotient $R(1)/R(0)$ into cell M8: **= M7/M6**, generating the value 0.5

12. Enter the formula $x[n] - a \cdot x[n - 1]$ into cell C10, using the Excel expression: **= C5 − $M8*B5**. This results in $d[0] = 512$.

13. Drag the formula from cell C10 to cell L10, producing the other difference signal samples, $d[n]$, which all have the value 0

14. Program the formula for the normalized prediction error into cell M11: **= SUMSQ (C10:L10)/SUMSQ(C5:L5)**. This gives us the value 0.75.

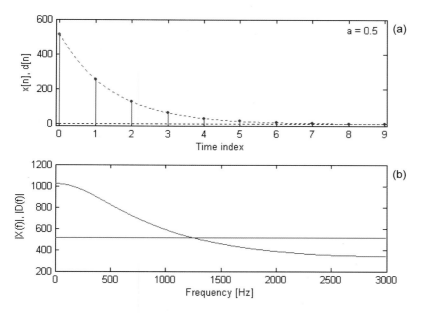

Figure 14–17   Input and output signals of first-order prediction with filter coefficient $a = \frac{1}{2}$: **(a)** waveforms and **(b)** spectra.

	A	B	C	D	E	F	G	H	I	J	K	L	M
1	Time index n	-1	0	1	2	3	4	5	6	7	8	9	
2	u[n]	0	512	0	0	0	0	0	0	0	0	0	
3	Filter coefficient												
4	a	- 1/2											
5	x[n]	0	512	-256	128	-64	32	-16	8	-4	2	-1	
6	R(0)												349525
7	R(1)												-174762
8	R(1) / R(0)												-0.50
9	Prediction filter												
10	d[n]		512	-0	0	-0	0	-0	0	-0	0	-0	
11	Normalized prediction error												0.75
12	k1 = R(1) / R(0)												-0.50
13	V = 1 - k1*k1												0.75

Figure 14–18   Calculation process for first-order prediction with filter coefficient $a = {}^{-}\frac{1}{2}$.

15. Take the value from M8 and enter it into cell M12: = **M8**

16. Put the Equation $1 - (k_1)^2$ into cell M13, using the Excel syntax: = **1 − M12*M12**. This also gives us the value 0.75.

First-Order Prediction with Negative Filter Coefficients

Figure 14–18 shows the Excel table for the example with filter coefficient $a = {}^{-1}/_2$. The easiest way to get this table is to copy the one from the previous example, and just change the filter coefficient value in cell B4.

The resonance filter produces the signal $x[n]$ in row 5, from the signal $u[n]$ in row 2. This time, the signal $x[n]$ constantly changes sign from one sample value to the next.

In contrast to the previous example, the autocorrelation value $R(1)$ also changes its sign, and therefore so does the quotient $R(1) / R(0)$ (i.e., the value of the filter coefficient in cell M8).

The prediction filter produces the signal $d[n]$ in row 10 from the signal $x[n]$ in row 5, thereby getting back the original signal $u[n]$. The normalized prediction error becomes the same as in the example with positive filter coefficients – both after the first calculation process, in cell M11, and after the second, in cell M13.

Figure 14–19a shows how the signal $x[n]$ oscillates about the zero line, and dies away. The spectrum in **Figure 14–19b** rises with increasing frequency, thereby reflecting the oscillating waveform.

Second-Order Prediction

The Excel table in **Fig. 14–20** shows the calculation procedure for the second-order prediction filter example, with filter coefficients $a_1 = 1$ and $a_2 = -1/2$.

Row 1 contains the time index, this time with values from -2 to 12. The test signal in row 2 has the value 64 at time $n = 0$, and is 0 everywhere else.

Cells B4 and B5 hold the filter coefficients $a_1 = 1$ and $a_2 = -1/2$. The second-order resonance filter uses these values to generate the output signal $x[n]$ in row 6.

Cells Q7 to Q9 contain the autocorrelation values $R(0)$, $R(1)$ und $R(2)$. The formulae in cells A10 to A12 use these values to calculate a denominator D and two numerators N_1 and N_2,

with the results appearing in cells Q10 to Q12. The filter coefficients a_1 and a_2 derive from these intermediate values, using the formulae $a_1 = N_1 / D$ and $a_2 = N_2 / D$.

Figure 14–21 shows the block diagram for second order prediction. The part with yellow background again represents the prediction filter. To get a sample of the difference signal $d[n]$,

1. Multiply the preceding input sample $x[n - 1]$ by filter coefficient a_1
2. Multiply the sample $x[n - 2]$ from two sample intervals earlier by the filter coefficient a_2
3. Sum the products, thus generating the estimate $y[n]$
4. Subtract the estimate $y[n]$ from the current input sample $x[n]$

Applying the second-order prediction to the signal $x[n]$ in the Excel table produces the difference signal $d[n]$ in row 16, and again the difference signal $d[n]$ exactly matches the test signal $u[n]$ in row 2.

As in the previous examples, it is possible to calculate the normalized prediction error from the individual samples of the signals $x[n]$ and $d[n]$, and to enter it into cell Q17. Cells Q18 and Q19 contain the reflection coefficients k_1 and k_2, calculated as follows:

$$k_1 = R(1)/R(0) \qquad \text{(Eq. 14-5)}$$

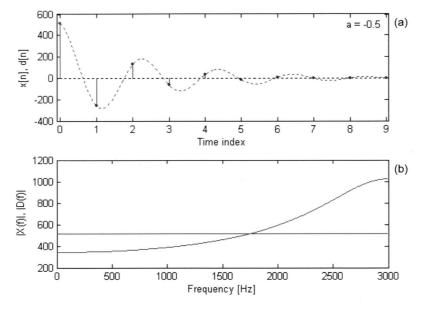

Figure 14–19 Input and output signals of first-order. Prediction with filter coefficient $a = -1/2$: **(a)** waveforms and **(b)** spectra.

A	B	C	D	E	F	G	H	I	J	K	L	M	N	O	P	Q
1 Time index n	-2	-1	0	1	2	3	4	5	6	7	8	9	10	11	12	
2 u[n]	0	0	64	0	0	0	0	0	0	0	0	0	0	0	0	
3 Filter coefficient																
4 a1	1															
5 a2	-1/2															
6 x[n]	0	0	64	64	32	0	-16	-16	-8	0	4	4	2	0	-1	
7 R(0)																9829
8 R(1)																6552
9 R(2)																1638
10 D = R(0)*R(0) - R(1)*R(1)																53680537
11 N1 = R(1)*R(0) - R(1)*R(2)																53667432
12 N2 = R(2)*R(0) - R(1)*R(1)																-26828802
13 N1 / D																1.00
14 N2 / D																-0.50
15 Prediction filter																
16 d[n]		64	0	0	0	0	0	0	0	0	0	0	0	0	0	
17 Normalized prediction error																0.42
18 k1 = R(1) / R(0)																0.67
19 k2 = N2 / D																-0.50
20 V = (1 - k1*k1)*(1 - k2*k2))																0.42

Figure 14–20 Calculation process for second-order prediction with filter coefficients $a_1 = 1$ and $a_2 = -\frac{1}{2}$.

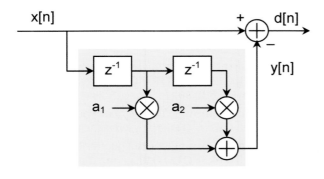

Figure 14–21 Block diagram of second-order prediction.

and

$$k_2 = a_2 \qquad \text{(Eq. 14-7)}$$

Using these values in the formula

$$V = (1 - (k_1)^2) \cdot (1 - (k_2)^2) \qquad \text{(Eq. 14-8)}$$

yields the prediction error $V = 0.42$ in cell Q20. The results in cells Q20 and Q17 are again identical.

Figure 14–22a shows how, in this example too, the signal $x[n]$ oscillates about the zero line, albeit with a lower frequency than in **Fig.**

14–19a. One oscillation lasts between eight and nine sampling intervals, that is, around 1.4 ms, taking into account the sampling rate of 6 kHz. This corresponds to a resonance frequency at 700 Hz in the spectrum, in accordance with the spectral peak in **Fig. 14–22b**.

To conclude, here are the individual calculation steps to create the Excel table in **Fig. 14–20**:

1. Enter the time index −2 into cell B1
2. Type the formula for this value plus one, into cell C1: = **B1 + 1**

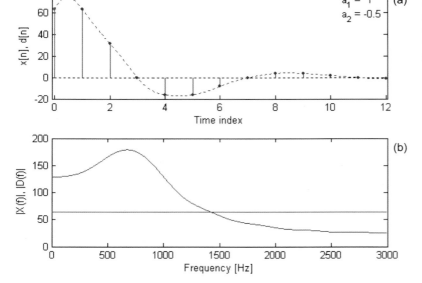

Figure 14–22   Input and output signals of second-order prediction with filter coefficients $a_1 = 1$ and $a_2 = -\frac{1}{2}$: **(a)** waveforms and **(b)** spectra.

3. Drag the formula from cell C1 to cell P1, producing the time indices up to $n = 12$

4. Enter the signal values $u[n]$ into cells B2 to P2: **64** in cell D2, **0** everywhere else

5. Put the filter coefficient values **1** and $^{-1}/_2$ into cells B4 and B5

6. Enter the initial value 0, for times $n = -2$ und $n = -1$, into cells B6 and C6

7. In cell D6, type the filter formula $u[n] + a_1 \cdot x[n - 1] + a_2 \cdot x[n - 2]$ using the Excel syntax: $= $ **D2+ \$B4*C6 + \$B5*B6**. This results in $x[0] = 64$.

8. Drag the formula from cell D6 to P6, generating the remaining sample values for signal $x[n]$

9. Enter the formula for the autocorrelation value $R(0)$ into cell Q7, using the Excel syntax: $= $ **SUMSQ(D6:P6)**. This gives us $R(0) = 9,829$.

10. Enter the formula for the autocorrelation value $R(1)$ into cell Q8, using the Excel syntax: $= $ **SUMPRODUCT(D6:P6,C6:O6)**. This gives us $R(1) = 6,552$.

11. Enter the formula for the autocorrelation value $R(2)$ into cell Q9, using the Excel syntax: $= $ **SUMPRODUCT(D6:P6,B6:N6)**. This gives us $R(2) = 1,638$.

12. Put the formula for the denominator D into cell Q10: $= $ **Q7*Q7 − Q8*Q8**; resulting in $N = 53,680,537$

13. Put the formula for the numerator N_1 into cell Q11: $= $ **Q8*Q7 − Q8*Q9,** resulting in $Z_1 = 53,667,432$

14. Put the formula for the numerator N_2 into cell Q12: $= $ **Q9*Q7 − Q8*Q8,** resulting in $Z_2 = -26,828,802$

15. Put the formula for the quotient N_1 / D into cell Q13: $= $ **Q11/Q10**, giving the value 1

16. Put the formula for the quotient N_2 / D into cell Q14: $= $ **Q12 / Q10**, giving the value -0.5

17. Enter the formula $x[n] - a_1 \cdot x[n - 1] - a_2 \cdot x[n - 2]$ into cell D16, using the Excel syntax: $= $ **D6 − \$Q13*C6 − \$Q14*B6**. This results in $d[0] = 64$.

18. Drag the formula from cell D16 to cell P16, generating the remaining sample values for the difference signal $d[n]$, all with the value 0

19. Type the formula for the normalized prediction error into cell Q17: $= $ **SUMSQ(D16:P16)/ SUMSQ(D6:P6)**. This gives the value 0.42.

20. Enter the formula for the quotient $R(1) / R(0)$ into cell Q18: $= $ **Q8 / Q7**, resulting in $k_1 = 0.67$

21. Take the value from cell Q14 and enter it into cell Q19: $= $ **Q14**

22. Enter the Equation $(1 - (k_1)^2) \cdot (1 - (k_2)^2)$ into cell Q20, using the Excel syntax: = **(1 − Q18*Q18)*(1 − Q19*Q19)**. This also results in the value 0.42.

◆ Summary

In this chapter, we explored autocorrelation and prediction. In the first section, we calculated the autocorrelation coefficient. Practical examples then demonstrated that it is possible to recognize whether or not a signal is periodic – and if so, what the period is.

In the second section, we familiarized ourselves with the mathematical background to prediction. First, we analyzed resonance filters. They change a signal with a flat spectrum in such a way that the spectrum of the output signal rises with frequency, falls, or contains a resonance. The analysis then showed how to derive the filter coefficients from the samples of these output signals.

Next, the focus was on how to transform the resonance filter into a prediction filter. Using the derived filter coefficients, prediction works in exactly the opposite way to the resonance filter, thus making it possible to reconstruct the signal that served as the input signal to the resonance filter in the first place.

Finally, the analysis showed how to calculate the normalized prediction error in two different ways. The first way was by taking individual sample values from both the input signal to the prediction filter and the difference between the predicted signal and the input signal. The second way was to calculate directly from suitable filter coefficients, in other words, without calculating either the output signal from the prediction filter, or the difference signal.

References

Baken, R.J., and Orlikoff, R.F. (2000). Clinical Measurement of Speech and Voice. Clifton Park, NY: Thomson Delmar Learning.

Chu, W.C. (2003). Speech coding algorithms: Foundation and evolution of standardized coders. Hoboken, NJ: Wiley-IEEE.

Goldberg, R.G, and Riek, L. (2000). A practical handbook of speech coders. Boca Raton, FL: CRC Press.

Greenberg, S., Popper, A.N., and Ainsworth, W.A. (2004). Speech processing in the auditory system. New York/Heidelberg/Berlin: Springer.

MacDonald, M. (2005). Excel: The missing manual. Sebastopol, CA: O'Reilly Media.

Padmanabhan, K., Ananthi, S., Vijayarajeswaran, R. (2003). A practical approach to digital signal processing. New Delhi, India: New Age International.

Vaton, S., Chonavel, T., and Ormrod, J. (2002). Statistical signal processing: Modelling and estimation. New York/Heidelberg/Berlin: Springer.

Wade, G. (1994). Signal coding and processing. New York: Cambridge University Press.

Zaknich, A. (2005). Principles of adaptive filters and self-learning systems. New York/Heidelberg/Berlin: Springer.

Zölzer U., Amatriain X., Arfib D., Evangelista G., Keiler F., Loscos A., Rocchesso D., Sandler M., Serra X., Todoroff T., Bonada J., De Poli G., and Dutilleux P. (2002). DAFX – Digital audio effects. Hoboken, NJ: John Wiley & Sons.

15

How Everything Fits Together

For most readers this book is like a journey—a tour leading from well known to unknown, from easy to difficult. This statement essentially holds for all those who have come across digital signal processing (DSP) for the first time. From chapter to chapter, the trend was from general to specific, from concrete to abstract. Now, it is time to summarize and focus on how all the pieces fit together.

The human brain stores knowledge in an associative network. Text, on the other hand, has a linear structure. Conveying knowledge thus requires serializing cognition into a sequence of thoughts. As you read a book, you absorb thought after thought; largely, you are left on your own to establish context. Our discussion here will point out how various topics in the book relate to each other. The sections in this chapter thus cover

1. *Retrospect*: summarizes in very broad outline what the three parts of the book presented before

2. *Hearing impairment and signal processing schemes*: recapitulates topics discussed at various places in the book and shows how they relate to major issues of hearing impairment

3. *Complexity of wide dynamic range compression* (*WDRC*): reviews the requirements to WDRC systems, enumerates the implementation options, and evaluates how the sound pressure level affects performance

In a book of moderate size, only a selection of all hearing aid topics can be described. The intent was to present the outstanding DSP features. Besides them, there are admittedly many more features – expansion or data logging, to name just two examples. Expansion is about how to set the compression characteristic for low sound pressure levels; it is the inverse of compression, actually, and results in applying less gain to low-level noise. Data logging, on the other hand, deals with storing data during hearing aid use, for later retrieval and evaluation. Although interesting in themselves, both features are good examples of why they are omitted from the book: they are simply not relevant to our understanding of the essential DSP features.

◆ Retrospect

My motivation behind this book was the technological change from analog to digital signal processing. The digital hearing instruments have displaced their analog predecessors on most markets, but many topics are still the same today as they were decades ago. This is what I covered in Part I of the book: the anatomy and functionality of the ear, acoustic signals, hearing impairment, and the basic strategy to overcome hearing loss; that is, to amplify the acoustic signals to make them again audible to a hearing-impaired person.

In Part II of the book I discussed how digital hearing instruments differ from the analog ones. First, they realize signal amplification in a different way—not all of them in a totally different way, but there are unparalleled options, such as processing in segments with Fourier transforms or using controllable filters, for example. Second, digital technology facilitates additional adaptive processing features: acoustic directionality, noise reduction, feedback cancellation, and signal classification.

The discussion in Part II, however, shifted only gradually to the digital signal representation. The focus was on how the desired effects come about. To this end, it was usually possible to explain how the algorithms work without stressing the character of the signals. There were exceptions, of course, where the digital nature of the signals was important: calculating running minima and maxima with noise reduction, for example, or the self-adjusting update mechanism in acoustic directionality and in feedback cancellation.

It is only in Part III that we closely examined digital signal processing – in two ways actually: first, numerous illustrations showed how to process a signal in segments, using the Fourier transform. Second, performing arithmetic with series of numbers provided insight into the basics of DSP. The numerical examples highlighted several aspects: filtering with finite impulse response (FIR) and infinite impulse response (IIR) filters, using a look-up table, measuring the sound pressure level, determining periodicity with autocorrelation, and estimating the gross shape of spectra with linear prediction.

◆ Hearing Impairment and Signal Processing Schemes

This section deals with five top issues regarding hearing impairment.

1. Sensorineural hearing loss accounts for the vast majority of all losses.

2. Understanding speech in noise is a major concern.

3. Noise of all kind is inconvenient.

4. Music should have a brilliant sound.

5. An occluded ear canal is annoying.

Now, let us review how the topics discussed in the book relate to these issues.

Sensorineural Hearing Loss

Measuring hearing loss involves finding the minimum sound pressure level of pure tones that an individual can just perceive. In general, hearing loss exhibits enormous variation in type, degree,

and configuration. In particular, a sensorineural hearing loss causes abnormal loudness growth. Band-limited noise signals usually serve as stimuli for measuring the loudness growth function.

Digital hearing aids offer wide dynamic range compression to compensate for sensorineural hearing loss; some hearing impaired persons, however, prefer linear amplification despite their abnormal loudness growth. In this case, a hearing aid usually activates compression only as a means of limiting very loud signals.

Prescribed target gain serves as a starting point only; the audiologist relies on speech audiometry to assess hearing as well as select and fit hearing aids.

In setting hearing aid gain, the fitting software considers the additional factors that amplify or attenuate sound on its path from the free field to the tympanic membrane. With increasing degree of hearing loss, more gain is needed and the tendency for acoustic feedback increases. In this case, feedback cancellation acts to prevent a hearing aid from howling.

Speech in Noise

Adaptive acoustic directionality is the best that digital hearing aids offer to improve understanding speech in noise. Assuming the desired signal source to be in the viewing direction, the processing scheme attenuates sounds approaching from the sides or rear. In practice, reverberation limits the benefit of acoustic directionality, making it necessary for a hearing aid user to stay close to the sound source of interest.

Sound classification may prove useful in automatically activating acoustic directionality and suitable gain settings in difficult listening situations. Calculating signal attributes and evaluating them, sound classification aims at telling everyday acoustic signals apart.

Noise

Noise reduction exploits the degree of modulation present in separate frequency bands to selectively pass or attenuate portions of an acoustic signal. As a result, such processing schemes are effective in suppressing monotonic noise, but fail in cases where a noise signal contains considerable modulation. Sound classification presents a more recent approach to overcome these shortcomings.

Music

Gain settings aiming at maximum speech intelligibility may prove less favorable to the sound of music. Moreover, noise reduction also adversely affects music that exhibits only little modulation. Sound classification is the best a digital hearing aid can offer to automatically assign separate music processing – or alternatively, a separate program that a hearing aid user can select manually.

Occluded Ear

Open fittings are popular among the various hearing aid styles because they avoid the occlusion effect. Nevertheless, there are also disadvantages – as with large vents. The signal path from the receiver to the microphone attenuates the amplified signal little, requiring feedback cancellation to accomplish more.

As the sound from the free field enters the ear canal more easily, there is also a risk of compromising the effects of acoustic directionality and noise reduction.

◆ Complexity of Wide Dynamic Range Compression

The complexity of WDRC systems derives from two factors.

1. Sensorineural hearing loss depending on frequency and sound pressure level
2. Sound pressure level representing a delicate quantity

Dependency Upon Frequency and Sound Pressure Level

The frequency-dependency of hearing loss calls for a flexible filter to provide sufficient gain shaping. The level-dependency tightens this requirement: the filter's gain curve must flexibly adapt as the sound pressure-level changes. For analog designers there was no way to come up with a filter that would satisfy these requirements. However, digital technology made it possible, in two versions actually: the controllable lattice filter and the controllable FIR filter.

Analog technology instead introduced multiband and multichannel systems. Digital technology added further options to band-splitting systems, but also provided a totally different scheme: segment-wise processing with Fourier transforms. Although not shown in the book, the Fourier transform also functions as a building block for advanced digital band-splitting systems.

Sound Pressure Level

The sound pressure level acts as the control variable in a WDRC system. At any point, the compression characteristic translates the current signal level into the amount of gain to apply to the signal.

The specifications for sound level measurement leave the question open as to what interval length is suitable for averaging. Objectives in this respect differ largely among various hearing instruments.

Measuring a running sound pressure level includes low-pass filtering to calculate an average. The low-pass filter produces a decaying, sliding observation window, and its length depends on the filter coefficient in the low-pass filter. The time constant of the whole WDRC system actually results from the filter coefficient, and the filter structure needs some refinement to produce smooth, accurate measurement values.

The averaging process causes the sound pressure level to lag the acoustic signal, giving rise to signal overshoots and thus calling for synchronization. Moreover, short time constants interact with the traditional multichannel WDRC structure to cause a loss of spectral contrast. On the other hand, ChannelFree processing combines with measuring an instantaneous sound pressure level, providing a distortion-free performance.

◆ Summary

In this chapter my aim was to establish context and to briefly review the topics discussed in the text. The focus was on showing how the various topics and processing schemes relate to major issues of hearing impairment. And finally, we recalled the subtle aspects that make WDRC a more intricate matter than one would believe at first glance.

Index